A NEW DAWN RISING

One Woman's Spiritual Odyssey

Teresita,
Best wishes
on your journey

Dawn Koh

Published by:
Zion Publishing
24040 Camino del Avion, Suite A166
Monarch Beach, CA 92629
Phone: 949-493-9382

ISBN: 0-9670201-0-7
Library of Congress Catalog Card Number: 99-93686

Printed in the United States of America
10 9 8 7 6 5 4 3 2 1

Though this story is true to the best of the author's memory, names have been changed to insure the protection of privacy.

To my children

Acknowledgments

Many people helped support me through this journey. My greatest thanks and appreciation goes to my husband, Philip, who had the strength and patience to hold our world together while my individual world fell apart. I appreciated you Philip, and all the ways you show me that you care. To my children, who have given me the honor of raising them, and who have helped to raise me, thanks for your patience, love and unconditional hugs and kisses. You are my greatest blessing.

To my friends, who watched, listened and listened again — you all know who you are, and I thank you. My thanks to Cheryl LaBarre for being there before, during and after. I appreciate you and our friendship beyond measure. And to my editors, Judith Searle of the editorial company, and my dear friends Alison Urbank and Lori Miller, your input and encouragement brought out the best in this story.

Prologue

In 1992 the spirit of a woman began to enter my life. At the time I was a wife, mother of three young children, and a part-time executive handling the financial matters of the growing computer company my husband and I founded shortly after college. I was not religious, by nature rebellious, and generally skeptical about supernatural events. By my own admission, I was not the kind of person I thought would be likely to receive a spiritual calling of the magnitude I came to experience.

The compelling events that followed led me on a three year journey. During that time my perception of the woman's spirit changed from an external perception of something around me, to the internal embodiment, and recognition that it was my own spirit connected to a spirit much greater than me.

This spontaneous transformation in consciousness came about through a difficult, turbulent and humbling process. I was often frightened, depressed, and then divinely inspired to continue down a path that taught me about my capacity to love, while releasing the debilitating effects of childhood trauma. To this extent it is a journey of personal healing. Yet this emotional, mental and physical clearing was the means to a greater gift – a spiritual message of a new beginning I was asked to give to others.

Chapter 1

I sat in the small lobby of Anne Myers' office staring at a tea table pushed up against the terracotta grass-cloth wall. Piano solos playing from a ceiling speaker glazed over the heavy silence. Down the narrow hall were four dark oak doors, all of them shut. I dropped my head back on the worn stuffed chair. How did my life lead me here, to a psychotherapist's office that felt like a dead end to a promising road?

The feeling in my chest flared; the heavy pull, the spiraling, comet-like energy that no one could diagnose. It had been six months since it started. And the ceaseless, foreign sensations were exhausting my body, keeping me up at night sweating and twitching, coursing through my veins like an alarm signaling *it was time* There was no logical reason, no medical explanation. And my intuition that the spiraling energy was trying to tell me something, that I was receiving some kind of a spiritual calling, was difficult for even me to believe. After all, I was a businesswoman, a borderline agnostic, a Republican — what would God want with me?

I closed my eyes, my thoughts jetting with the daily concerns for my three young children. Were they getting a bath? Was the baby crying? Was my husband home to relieve the housekeeper? I took a deep breath and let out a long, even deeper sigh. *I really don't want to be here.*

A moment of silence, a fleeting thought to leave, then my mother's southern laughter came crashing through my thoughts, advice I'd heard for everything from a bad dream to appendicitis. *You're fine. It's all in your head. You just need something to do to keep you busy.* My father's stern, deep voice chimed in after hers, so ingrained in my mind I thought it to be my own. *Dawn, there are people in the world with real problems, and you're not one of them.*

I heard a door open and footsteps came down the hall. I sat up straight, my darkening blonde hair falling onto the broad-padded shoulders of my silk navy-blue business suit, my athletic body worn down to fair skin on stubborn bones.

A sable-haired woman in her late thirties appeared. "Hi, are you Dawn?"

"Yes."

"My name is Anne. Why don't you come back to my office?"

I stared at her before I stood up. She was a short, medium-built woman wearing a pink and white striped cotton dress that somehow didn't suit her angular face, light olive-tone skin and long, thick wavy hair. She teetered nervously on her toes. It was an awkward moment. I pulled myself up to greet her, stood tall, straightened my shoulders, and walked down the hall before her.

We walked back into a small but comfortable office. A narrow walnut desk was pushed up against one wall, a rose-colored couch against the other. And an overstuffed chair stood in front of a large bay window that looked through an aspen tree in full bloom. The room was decorated in soft florals and the walls painted a warm shade of pink. I tossed my keys on the end table and sat down on the couch.

"Would you like a cup of tea or coffee?"

"No, thank you."

She picked up a tea bag and bounced it up and down in a cup of hot water.

"You said on the phone that you were referred by Dr. Barns. What seems to be the trouble?"

Our eyes met and Anne's shoulders let down. She took a deep breath and released it softly. I sat back and rattled off my business history first, the rapid growth of our computer company, the Orange County Woman Entrepreneur of the Year finalist award I had received a few years back. I wanted her to know I was accomplished before admitting I had a problem. Then, I told her about my symptoms, quickly glazing over the unexplainable energy flaring in my chest and focusing on the more recent, tangible feelings of emptiness, depression and fatigue.

"So there you have it," I said. "What's your diagnosis?"

Anne took a sip of her tea and looked across the distance between us warmly, almost enchanted. "I don't give diagnoses. I don't know what's wrong with you any more than you do."

I looked at my keys and thought about leaving.

"Dawn, your mind is trying to tell you something, and it's using your body to get your attention. It will take some time and dedication on both our parts to determine what's causing your symptoms."

"How much time?"

"With weekly sessions it could take months, maybe years."

"Years? You've got to be kidding."

"Therapy takes time."

"What's the short cut?"

She smiled and her eyes continued to soften. "It sounds to me like you've put a great deal of time into avoiding your problems. If you're willing to invest half that time into solving them, you will have your short cut."

Her tone was disarming, and I didn't want to be disarmed.

"How long have you been a therapist?"

"About three years."

"Have you ever been in therapy yourself?"

"Yes."

"What for?"

"I had an eating disorder."

She didn't look over-weight, or under nourished.

"Are you married?"

"Yes, I've been married for...let's see...about thirteen years."

"Any kids?"

"My husband has a child from his first marriage."

"You never had children of your own?"

"No, we decided not to."

"Was that difficult?"

"Yes, I think about it at times, but there are so many adult children in the world who need help, I decided that being a therapist was where my energy could provide the best service."

She took another sip of tea. She was holding up to my questioning better than I thought she would.

"What did you do before you were a therapist?"

"I was an editor for a magazine. My undergraduate degree is in journalism."

"Really, where did you go to school?"

"It was a school up in Sacramento. You've probably never heard of it."

"Sacramento State?" I asked.

"Yes. You've heard of it?"

"I went to school there when I was a freshman. My first major was in journalism."

"How come you changed?" she asked.

Feeling more comfortable, I shared with her that I didn't do well in my journalism class. I had grown up in La Jolla, a small beach community in Southern California. It was my first time away from home and I missed the ocean. In La Jolla, just a few miles from my home, I could stand out on a breezy cliff and look out to sea. It was like standing at the edge of the world. The hard black pavement had finally came to an end and the vast immortal body of passionate blue water rolled in front of me like an invitation to eternity. Without the sight of the ocean, I felt drained. The land had closed me in and it showed up in my schoolwork. My articles were returned as if my professor had bled on them. And the criticism, without any praise, triggered a shame so deep it felt as if it could destroy me.

"At the end of the semester I moved back to San Diego, started selling real estate, and majored in business at San Diego State."

"That's funny," she said. "I did my graduate work in San Diego, not far from La Jolla."

She took another sip of her tea. I had exhausted my questions and was now intrigued by her presence. She felt familiar, although I knew I'd never met her. "Dawn, what is it you would like to achieve in therapy? Is there a goal you would like to accomplish?"

I thought about it for a moment.

"Yes." I said, "Peace of mind. Do you think that's possible?"

"Absolutely."

"You mean to tell me that I can really find peace in this world?"

"Yes. You absolutely can."

"Will I have to take drugs? Because I'm not interested in trading symptoms for side effects."

"Have you taken medication before?"

I told her that in my early twenties I had been put on a medication for panic attacks, unexpected rushes of adrenaline that made me dizzy, breathless, and often consumed me with a dread of being killed that sometimes lasted days.

"The only thing worse than the panic attacks," I said, "was the curl-up-and-die depression that hit me a few weeks after I started the medication."

She nodded. "You don't have to worry, medication won't be necessary."

If she didn't know what was wrong with me, how could she be so sure about a cure?

"You sound so sure about this. How do you know if I'm even capable of having a peaceful mind?"

"I guess you're just going to have to trust me on this one. But I guarantee you, if you're willing to do the work, you will find a peace you never knew existed."

I didn't know if I believed her, but she was offering more hope than anybody I had ever met.

"Okay," I said, "for the sake of argument, let's say you help me find out what's causing my anxiety. There's still this other thing that happens to me that drives me crazy."

"What's that?"

"Sometimes I can't feel my body. I can still move, but I can't feel my skin, my body sensations go numb and my awareness rolls up in my head. Then it's like I'm seeing the world through a tunnel, almost like I'm detached from my body. It's very frightening and it can sometimes last for hours."

"What you're describing is called dissociation."

"There's a name for it?"

"Yes, many people suffer the same symptom. Do you lose time frames?"

I leaned forward, hoping she would offer more clarity.

"Sometimes when people dissociate, they lose blocks of time. Suddenly, the last memory they had was yesterday morning, or last week."

"No," I said. "I just lose the feel of my senses, but I don't black out or lose my sense of time. Why do people dissociate?"

"It's a survival technique. People experience it when they're in a bad accident or take a hard fall. It's the mind's way of protecting itself from a traumatic experience."

"So why do I do it?"

"I don't know. I presume that's one of the reasons you're here."

Her legs were lightly crossed, her face softened by light coming through the window behind her. She was smart but gentle—too gentle to handle me.

"Dawn, can you tell me a little more about the energy in your chest? What it feels like and when it started?"

"I woke up into it about eight months ago, and since then it's been like I'm in a fight with an invisible force. I want to keep on with my life and this force in my body wants me to so something else."

Anne looked as if she was absorbing my words, I felt understood and continued. "And it's insistent. I know this might sound strange, but it feels as if I'm receiving some sort of a calling."

"Do you have any idea what kind of calling?"

"No, it just feels big, much bigger than me."

"I'm sure it is." She put down her tea and leaned forward. The distance between us had narrowed and the air around us felt good, warm. "Do you have any more questions you want to ask me before we wrap up?"

"No."

She stood up and handed me a large white information folder that was sitting on the edge of her desk. I tucked the folder under my arm and then she extended her hand, the gesture seeming too formal for the mood.

"I don't know what your plans are," she said, "but by some leap of faith you've come here. It's up to you if you want to follow it."

Her words were spoken through her eyes, a stare I didn't break. A leap of faith had brought me to her. My doctor had given me her business card six months ago and her name had been haunting me ever since. But still, a nagging doubt kept me from making another appointment. There was something incongruent about her. When she stood, her shoulders moved down instead of back, as if she thought she was smaller than she was. And the awkwardness of some of her gestures made me feel she was more comfortable in her chair as therapist, than out of it.

My husband Philip and I met on a foursquare court in the seventh grade. I was in my hip-hugger jeans, wearing a backwards baseball cap, fiercely trying to reclaim my championship title from Lori Krug, my childhood friend who beat me at everything from pitching pennies to arm wrestling. Phil was standing in line with a group of his friends, gangly-limbed practical jokers who did well in science but didn't act like it.

Back then we didn't say much to each other. I was more interested in business than boys. I had saved enough money from a summer job to buy three coin-operated washing machines that my dad helped me place in one of the apartment buildings he owned. Once a month we'd take a pillowcase down to the building and empty the coins out of the machines. Dad would tell me to go put the money in the bank. Instead, I'd ride my bike down to the local broker and buy stock in small computer companies based solely on the color of their logo.

Phil was more interested in joking around, sneaking into girls' bedrooms and duct taping their stuffed animals to the ceiling. We didn't have much in common back then, but still, I remembered seeing something sweet in him. Or maybe it was sad. He didn't talk about it, but everybody in school knew Phil's dad had died. Some people said it was from heart disease. The kids in his neighborhood just said he drank too much.

His mother remarried a few years later, and by the time we started dating in my first year of high school, he had two stepbrothers and a baby sister who Philip cared for after school. That's what began to attract me to him. He could be loud, sometimes obnoxious, and occasionally drop-down drunk. But he loved children, and he was good with them.

Philip and I married the year after college, just after starting our computer service company, ICON. The years since then had been good. There was the success of our corporation, a few tranquil vacations to Mexico, and the births of our three children. Each labor had its unique difficulty. Each birth ended in Philip cutting the umbilical cord and tearfully lifting the baby to my breasts.

Now, it had been a year since our last child was born, and the air in our house was changing—the spiraling ball of energy in my chest more insistent. Each morning, it was becoming more difficult to get out of bed. And since I'd met Anne, each night just before nodding off to a restless sleep, a thought would push through my mind.

Anne Myers, she will help you.

A month later, I returned to begin therapy.

I sat in the small lobby staring at the wooden tea table. On the hour, Anne came out to greet me. We walked into her office, more comfortable than before. She offered me tea, and I accepted.

"I'm glad you came back," she said.

"I get the feeling I'm supposed to be here."

"Do you have premonitions?"

"I sometimes feel attracted to people I'm supposed to know, or things I'm suppose to do."

"Maybe you're psychic."

"No, I'm psycho. That's why I'm here."

She smiled and picked up her pen.

"If it's all right, I'd like to start by taking a family history."

She asked me about Philip, then the names and ages of our children. I told her Erica, Michael and Samantha were one, two and a half, and five.

"Any problems with the kids?"

"No. So far all three of them have had fun, easy-going dispositions."

She smiled. "Are your parents still living?"

"Yes. We see them about once a month. They get along well with Philip and the kids and we enjoy being around them."

"Do you have any brothers or sisters?"

"Three. My brother, James, is three years older, Mark is two years younger, and my sister Kris is four years younger than I am."

She turned over a page in her notebook, as if the questions were about to become more difficult.

"Could you describe your relationship with your parents as a child?"

I sat up in my chair and stared at her.

"Anne, I'm here because this energy in my chest is telling me I have to do something in the future. I don't really want to waste time talking about my past."

She lowered her pen and looked at me, gently. "I believe you do have something to do. And I also believe we need to understand who we are, and how our lives have affected us, in order to discover and fulfill our life calling."

Again, I felt unarmed by her, as if every time I drew my sword, she would tenderly remove it with words I could understand. With compassion I had not known. I nodded and revisited the question.

The thought of my childhood always thrust me back to dinnertime, to the evenings my brothers and I came in from playing outside with the neighbors to a house transformed from the shambles in which we left it. In my mind I could see the rust-colored shag carpeting that ran through our three-bedroom home cleared of toys, clothing and animals. The teak coffee table between the gold chenille couches where our half-finished glasses of milk usually sat, was cleared and dusted, and the white walls and oil paintings were now softened by the waning light that came through the windows on each side of the fireplace.

My mother, a beautiful green-eyed, dark-olive skinned woman who seemed to enjoy spending her days taking care of my baby sister, ironing my father's shirts and feeding whoever walked into the house, now stood in the kitchen freshly showered, made-up, and trying as best she could to look like Jacqueline Kennedy stepping off the page of a magazine.

My dad walked through the door sometime after six, his thinning black hair still neatly combed back, his tie loosened, his shoulders drooping as if the long days at his architecture firm were somehow designed to kill him. My mother greeted him with a soft, sensuous kiss, and the sides of his mouth turned up before he shrugged off her affection as an invasion, or an embarrassment.

"Come on, kids, dinner's ready!" Mom said as she grabbed the pot-holders to pull the pop-up biscuits out of the oven.

We ran to claim our seats around a Danish teak table, all of us trying to sit by Dad, me getting to the chair first. After Dad sat down, Mom served, then she went around the table and asked each of us about our day. Nothing very exciting was shared, so to liven up the dinner, my brothers and I resorted to teasing, tripping up my mother's presentation by not-so-accidentally knocking over the salt shaker. To reverse the inevitable bad luck, Mom hurled herself across the table, grabbed the shaker, and tossed salt over each shoulder. We laughed, Dad ignored it and Mom attempted to regain her cool.

"Better the devil you know," she said in her fading southern accent.

Over dessert, Dad's grunts gave way to words and an occasional whole sentence. In the lighter moments, when he looked up from his plate and the air between us didn't feel so tense, I searched for something good to say, something I'd done that would make him proud — or make him laugh.

"They were normal," I said to Anne. "My mom wasn't really a factor in my life. We're closer now that I've had children, but when I was young there was no real connection. I have always felt like I pretty much raised myself."

"What about your father?"

I laughed, though I didn't know why. If I really felt like opening up to her, I would have told her that my dad was the one who raised me. We had something special. A connection I never had with my mother. He was the one who went to my tennis games, took me to work with him on Saturdays, and was always interested in what I was doing as long as it was productive. We'd laugh at jokes nobody else in the family would get, and talked about world events nobody else in the family was interested in. As a child, he was everything to me. He was my hero.

My dad grew up in Ohio, in a strict German Catholic home, married my mom the year he graduated from college, and moved to San Diego to take a draftsman's job at an architecture firm. A few years later he designed a home to fit on a long, narrow lot. The design won him an award and gave him enough money to start his own building company. I was always proud of him for that. Not just because he worked hard and he was successful because of it, but because he did it with a handicap.

When he was a teenager his right hand had been badly deformed in a fireworks accident. What remained didn't look like a hand at all, but one mangled hook-shaped finger coming out of a disfigured dome. In high school, he had to learn how to write using his left hand, and my grandmother said he practiced every night until he was strong enough to get into architecture school. I have often thought our family was built on that story—or at least I was.

I looked up at Anne. It seemed like everything that I had worked for in my life, I had worked for to make my dad proud. But things had changed. He hadn't spoken to me much since I married Philip. He liked Phil, but I had a strange sense that my marriage somehow betrayed him.

"My dad helped me out," I said. "When he approved of what I was doing he would help out financially, give me some encouragement and then make sure I worked my butt off to make it happen. And when he didn't approve—he just stopped talking to me."

"That must have hurt."

"No, not really. I wasn't affected by my parents."

She paused, looking at me like she wanted me to say more. I had nothing more I wanted to say.

"Did your parents have a good relationship?"

"Yes. Occasionally I'd hear them bickering, but for the most part they seemed to get along."

"Did either one of them use drugs or alcohol?"

I hesitated. "Does wine count?"

"Last time I checked."

"My mother's a wine drinker."

"Was it excessive?"

Excessive. From about the time I was in the third grade on, it was. After she ran the car pools, did the shopping and baked a batch of cookies, she spent her afternoons with a couple of her girlfriends eating cheese spreads that came out of plastic containers and drinking white wine from a jug poured into crystal glasses. The void of inebriation, a stupidity that sent me into a silent fury, glazed her eyes for the rest of the evening.

"At times," I said.

"Did that bother you?"

"I don't know. I guess I told her to stop a few times."

"And did she?"

I smirked. "Yes. She stopped drinking out of wine glasses and started drinking out of coffee mugs."

"How did that make you feel?"

"Like the wine was more important than I was."

"That's a very sad statement. Why did you say it with a smile?"

"It wasn't that big a deal. Anyway, like I said, I raised myself."

She tilted her head as if she didn't quite believe me, then wrote something down on her note pad. "That's interesting that as a little girl you made the decision to raise your self. Why do you think you made it?"

"I don't trust people."

"Why not?"

"People are selfish. They only care about themselves, so it's always been safer to stay on my own."

"What about your husband and children?"

"I take care of my kids—they don't take care of me. And Phil and I are very self-sufficient. We make good partners, but we do just as well on our own."

"What about your needs?"

"I don't have needs."

She put down her pen and looked at me. Her eyes were large, a muted blue with a gaze more loving than perceptive.

"Can you remember the last time you got upset or cried?"

"No, and there are two things about me that you should probably know. I don't cry, and I don't throw up."

"You've never thrown up?"

"Once, but that was because my appendix burst."

"It sounds like you have a great deal of self control."

"It's better than losing it."

She looked at me, then drew something on a piece of paper and raised her clipboard to show me:

FEELING-SOBBING-CONTROLLING

"Dawn, at one point in your existence you were a feeling child, fully alive and in tune with your needs and emotions. Somewhere along the line, you were emotionally injured. If you were not safe to feel your pain, you began to control it, and by doing so you cut yourself off from the natural flow of your emotions. We all have needs, and denying their existence doesn't make them go away, it only stuffs them down to be dealt with later."

"So what? Everybody has problems. What's the point in wallowing in them?"

"The point is they are making you unhealthy, and if you don't care enough about yourself to do something about them, nobody is going to be able to help you." Her voice softened. "Dawn, you have no reason to trust me — you hardly know me. But with time you will need to let somebody in to help you deal with whatever is causing you so much pain."

I was feeling exposed and unusually comfortable with it. "Anne, there are people in the world with real problems. I don't feel I deserve the attention."

"Why don't you deserve it?"

"I don't know. I feel like I was born a bad person. I've always had a lot of guilt about the way I am."

"Can you explain that?"

"I've worked very hard in my life to prove that I'm a good person, but deep inside I feel like I've done something very wrong."

"I don't believe you're a bad person. And I don't for a minute believe you were a bad child."

"You don't?"

"No, I don't. But I think it's important to find out why you feel that way."

She was listening to me, and she wasn't laughing. Not the way my mother did — the non-believing chuckle she would give me whenever I told her I felt sick, or was afraid something terrible was about to happen me.

"I don't know if this is related," I said, "but there's something else that's been bothering me."

"We've got time."

I couldn't look at her, the embarrassment shrinking me as I sank into the couch, my toes turning in and crossing. Telling Anne about the feelings made them worse — the flush beneath my skin that opened every pore with a starvation for a woman's touch. An embrace that cradled me close to a breast. Soft round arms blanketing me in a thick fragrance of acceptance, love, protection.

"Did your mother ever hold you?" Anne asked.

"No, but that was my fault. She says she tried to give me affection but I wouldn't accept it. She said even when I was in a crib I would cry for hours and when she came in to hold me I pushed her away."

"Do you have any idea why?"

"No, I just remember I was always angry with her — for taking my younger brother's side every time we got in a fight. Or for lying to my father trying to make it sound as if she had us kids under control when she didn't. And," I said as I released a deep breath, "I was always trying to prove that I didn't need her. I guess I'm starting to regret that now. My body aches to be held like a child, but I'm thirty-two years old. It's a little late to be mothered."

There was a deep sadness in Anne's eyes. Either she felt the same pain, or she felt mine so deeply she could show me what it looked like.

"Dawn, I hear you blaming yourself for all of this. You were the one that pushed people away. You were the one that was a bad kid. Wasn't anybody responsible for you?"

"Yes, they were, but like I said, I made the decision to raise myself. I didn't want anybody's help, and I guess in a way, my behavior caused me to be neglected."

"Behavior doesn't cause our neglect," she said. "Neglect causes our behavior, and for you to make a decision at such a young age to be so totally independent, you had to somehow come to the conclusion that you were taking better care of yourself than anybody else in the house."

"Anne, I'm responsible for my own life. I don't want to dump this back on my parents."

"It's not necessary to dump it back on them. In fact, you don't ever have to talk to them about it. But for your own welfare, you need to become aware of what was their neglect and what was yours, and right now all I'm hearing is that, from the time you were just a little kid, you felt so powerful that you could push away the adults in your life who were supposed to care for you. And now that your childhood needs have surfaced, it's all your fault."

"That's what it feels like."

"How old is Samantha?"

"Five."

"If one of your children were not getting their basic needs met, would you blame it on the child?"

"No."

"Then you should have some compassion for yourself, because in essence, you are no different than your children."

No different from my children? I was completely different from my children. They were innocent, joyful, untainted by the world. I couldn't remember a time when I felt the same.

I looked over at Anne and her eyes shot down.

"Oh," she said as she jumped up from her chair. "Look at the time! I have to get going." She walked over to her desk and opened her scheduling book.

"Is the same time Tuesday okay for you?"

"Yes, that will be fine."

She put down her pen and turned toward me, her sweet, smoky perfume fragrance in the air. It was the first time our eyes had meet so close. We stood silent for a moment.

"Is it all right if I hug you?" she asked.

I smiled, flattered that she'd asked, more comfortable with the request than I would have thought. She held me till I pulled away. More than a brief moment and I would have felt awkward.

"Why don't you ask one of your friends to hold you," she said.

"No, I wouldn't be comfortable with that."

"How come?"

"I don't know. I guess I'm just not that kind of a person."

Anne encouraged me to start a journal and to begin by writing down some childhood memories and any feelings I could associate with them. I resisted the idea at first. I was still more interested in discovering what I was being called to do with my future than waste time with my past. But I wanted Anne to know I was willing to work, so after tucking the kids in one night, I walked into my nest—a loft above the dinning room. It was my hide-a-way: a small, taupe painted room with thick cream carpeting where I had carefully placed my old wooden desk, a white-feather daybed and a built-in book shelf that ran the length of the loft wall. Next to my desk and across from the bookshelf, a three-pane window looked out through the palm trees that encircled the brick patio and on to a small private golf course that nestled up against the sage-green foothills rising up beyond the view out my window.

I lay down on the bed and rested the journal across my chest. I didn't know what to write about. My childhood all seemed so normal. My mom took us to the beach all summer, cut up watermelon for all our friends, and laughed as childishly as we did as we spit out the black seeds from the melon, trying to get them to cling to each other's hair. And my dad was like everybody else's dad. He worked all week, made us do yard work with him on Saturday afternoons, and on Sundays he took us skin diving in our favorite cove.

I turned over and stared out the window. Then why was I so scared as a child? And why did I dissociate? I began to remember the first time it happened. I was five, maybe six-years-old. After dinner my mother had sent me to take a bath. I poured in the Mr. Bubble, stepped in the tub and pulled closed the green plastic curtain. I slid down in the bath till the warm water covered my ears, my white-blonde hair flooding on the bubbling surface, my toes barely long enough to touch the drain. Sinking deeper into the warm water's embrace my muscles began to let down.

I closed my eyes. Silence. Then, I heard the deep rapid pounding of my heart, thumping faster and harder as if it was running away. My eyes shot wide open. The tile walls looked as though they were moving. I jerk myself up, caught my breath, and looked down at the drops of water running down my arms. I couldn't feel them. My skin had gone numb, and my hands didn't feel attached to my body. I slapped my cheeks for a moment, then dug my thumbnail into the palm of my hand. I saw the sight of blood and I still felt nothing.

"Dawn are you still in there?" My mother spoke from behind the door. Her voice sounded like a distant call.

I jumped out of the tub, panting, covering my mouth so my mother wouldn't hear.

"I'm out," I yelled. My voice didn't sound as if it was my own. I dried off and put on my blue flannel pajamas, then headed for the back door to try and get some air. My mother passed me in the hall and grabbed me by the arm.

"Where are you running off to?"

"Nowhere."

"Then get in your room and put your clothes out for tomorrow. You kids are all going to bed by 7:30."

My two-year-old sister, Kristen, and I slept in twin beds in a small room across from the bathroom. Around 8:30 my mother put us to bed. She smiled through her tired, green eyes as she nestled Kristen into her covers, sang her a song and kissed her goodnight on the forehead. Then she came over to my bed. I straight-armed her before she could get near me.

"Don't touch me."

She chuckled. "Oh, Dawn, you're always trying to grow up so fast."

She turned off the light and I waited in the dark, nauseated, rolled up in my white cotton sheets chanting to myself that I wasn't going to throw up. When I heard my dad click off his light and release a deep sigh, I tiptoed across the carpet and crawled under the sheets to join Kristen in her bed. With her warm body wrapped in my arms, her soft brown hair against my cheeks, I prayed: *God, please keep our family together and some day make me safe.*

Chapter 2

nne and I spent the next month talking about my family. Things between us seemed to be clicking and it wasn't long before I was as comfortable with her as I had ever been with anybody. We'd spend the first few minutes of our sessions joking around, talking about current events or something amusing one of the kids had done. Then she'd pick up her pen and pull me back into my childhood.

One day she asked about my grandparents. I had only met my mother's parents once. I was in the third grade and my parents took us out of school for two weeks to drive back to West Virginia to spend Thanksgiving with our relatives.

The car trip started out as most of them did. We all piled in our wood paneled Ford station wagon. My brother, Mark, who was 18 months younger than I, crawled underneath me and went for my seat. I grabbed him by the back of his T-shirt and pulled his buzz haircut dome up to my shoulders. He shrilled like an Indian declaring battle, swung and rocketed his fist deep into my stomach. I dropped to the car floor, gasping to catch my breath. Without a word Dad grabbed Mark by the back of the neck and firmly sat him down in the small trundle seat that pulled up in the back. He asked if I was all right then directed me to seat in the middle. Mom climbed in with my little sister clinging around her neck, pretending she didn't see the incident. And my older brother, James, who had dark-skin like my mom and curly, brown hair like my sister, jumped in next to me.

To make sure I was alright he started to tickle me, smiling through light-blue eyes, one just a little lazier than the other. When he saw I was okay, he climbed to the back to make sure Mark was.

We drove mostly at night. Mom slept in the back with the other kids while I sat in the front and kept dad company. He taught me how to read the map, making up stories so I'd remember the names of the towns. Gila Bend, he said, was pronounced *Hila* and was named after a big lizard. And Albuquerque was Indian for *the place where the cops go to have donuts*.

As the night wore on, he taught me how to caculate time versus distance. And in the pre-dawn hours, I made a deal with him that if I stayed up until sunrise he'd have to buy me a piece of cherry pie for breakfast. Everybody in the back of the car was still asleep when the night sky turned red and a brillant gold sun peaked up over the foothills. Dad pulled off the freeway just outside of Little Rock, Arkansas into a small, road-side café with a wood-post fence lining a four car parking lot. The two of us went in and sat down at an old grey-specked counter. Dad had coffee. I had the best piece of cherry pie I'd ever eaten.

On the third day we drove through the gold and auburn trees that lined the Appalachian mountains and arrived in Hatfield Bottom, the town where Mom was raised, and where the Hatfields and McCoys once feuded over land. I felt transported in time. We pulled up to my grandparents' house, an old two-story building with outdoor plumbing and a porch that looked as though it had been through the Civil War.

My grandmother, a short round woman who had given birth to 16 children, the fourteenth being my mother, came out the chipped, white door with a smile that rose up to the dark puffy skin that folded under her eyes. She picked me up first, wrapped her portly arms around me and smothered me between her large sagging breasts. She then reached for my brothers, grabbing them at the same time as she kissed Kristen and mom.

"Oh, Ezra," she yelled to my grandfather. "Come on and see these kids."

My grandfather, a tall and stoic coal miner wearing a fresh pair of ironed over-alls, walked up from behind the house. Mom introduced him to James and Mark, and before he met Kristen, he turned to me and nodded.

"What can I get for you young lady?" His eyes shone like royal blue marbles.

"Nothing," I replied.

He stared at me as if I were a precious sight, something rare and sacred that he valued with an unspoken appreciation. For the rest of the week he treated me like royalty. When the rest of the kids were bathing together in an old wooden tub that sat on the back lawn, he insisted that I bathe alone. He made sure I was well fed and watched me closely, but from a distance. And many times that week I heard him tell my mom, "You need to take good care of that child."

Mom told me he treated me that way because of some superstition. I didn't believe in superstitions, but it felt good to be treated that way.

My grandmother died a few months after we left West Virginia and my grandfather died six months after her. I told Anne that I thought it was around that time when my mom's drinking became a problem. Anne seemed concerned about that. She wanted to know how I felt when I saw my mother with a glass of wine, or noticed she was impaired. But my memories of my mother half-asleep on the couch, directing me to do chores while I ignored her, didn't elicit much emotion for me, just a deepening depression. I felt like a sewer tank had ruptured in my system, polluting my body with toxins too dense to release with tears. All I wanted to do was sleep all day, and every time Anne hugged me good-bye, an embrace that was lasting a little longer each session, my depression seemed to worsen.

I walked into my next session with Anne desperate for relief. "You know," I said as I entered her office, "ever since I started to see you, my symptoms have gotten worse. Can't you do something about this?"

"I don't know. What symptoms are you referring to?"

My skin was painfully yearning to be held. My stomach churning from a childlike terror while my body was aching for a safe refuge.

"The need to be held by a woman is worse than ever. And worse than that is this feeling of dread, this anxiety, this feeling like I'm about to die."

Anne leaned forward as she looked into my eyes, her taupe-green silk blouse draped loosely over the thigh of her matching leggings.

"When you say you feel like your about to die, how do you experience that feeling?"

"With terror, a kind of hopeless panic. When I've had the feeling in the past, I associated it to my health. If the dread came with a headache, I thought I had a brain tumor that was going to kill me. If

I was overly fatigued when I felt the dread, I'd go into a panic thinking I had some fatal blood disease. But now I feel it every day. It's as if the fear of death is coming closer."

"Do you recall when the fear started?"

"It goes back as far as I can remember...maybe to when I was five or six years old."

"Did you ever tell your mother about it?"

"Yes, several times. But she told me I worried too much and either gave me some homespun cliché or suggested that I take up an art project or a musical instrument."

She shook her head and let out a deep sigh then leaned back in her chair and thought for a moment. "Have you ever heard of guided imagery?"

"No."

"Guided imagery is a technique used for achieving a state of focused concentration. It allows for more of the unconscious mind to come forward into conscious awareness."

"Sounds like hypnosis."

"It is a form a hypnosis. The difference is that in a guided imagery session the client leads the direction rather than the therapist."

"How do you do it?"

"You just close your eyes and take a few deep breaths. With your eyes closed, your mind will begin to focus inward and the breathing will help to keep you relaxed."

"Is that when you tell me to walk like a chicken?"

She wasn't amused. "Unfortunately, stage shows have made trance work out to be some kind of hocus pocus. But actually, it's a very effective tool to override severe fears and get a better understanding of the conflict that's going on underneath them."

"What kind of trance?"

"It's like meditation or biofeedback. All it is, is focused concentration."

"Will I remain conscious?"

"Yes. You will be conscious the entire time and you will always have control over your experience."

"Okay. If I'm in control, I'll give it a try."

I leaned back on the couch and closed my eyes. A stereo was playing a piano solo in the background. Anne turned down the music and spoke in a slightly lower pitch, a peaceful tone that made me feel almost safe. She gave me a few suggestions to breathe deeply and release muscle tension, and as she did I entered a state of relaxation similar to my feeling before I fall asleep. My mind was still awake, but I was no longer aware of my body.

"Dawn, I want you to imagine that there is a gold ring around the area of your heart. When you have that image, let me know."

I focused my concentration on the inside of my chest where a thick gold ring appeared surrounded by darkness.

"I see it."

"Good. Now with your thoughts, I want you to ask a child to appear, and when the child appears I want you to describe it to me."

Through the ring came an image of me as a five-year-old.

"I see her. It's me when I'm about five."

"Describe her to me. What she's wearing? What's her facial expression? Or tell me anything else you notice."

"She's wearing jeans and a black turtleneck. Her hair is blonde, about shoulder length, with long bangs pushed to the side of a face smudged with dirt. She is standing in the ring, staring at me with her pug nose slightly crunched up and her eyes squinting.

"What else do you notice about her?"

"She looks intense... perceptive. Not like a child... but like she's already grown up."

"Ask her if it's all right if we speak with her for a few minutes."

The image was strong. I could feel the intensity of my concentration on the child. With my thoughts I asked if she would speak with me. Without any conscious attempt on my part, the child answered.

Are you my mother?

"Anne, this child wants to know if I'm her mother."

"Tell her for now you will be."

Before I could respond, the child said, *I don't trust you* and ran out of the gold circle into the darkness.

"I lost her, Anne. She said 'I don't trust you' and then she ran away."

"She's just a child. Go get her."

After a few seconds the child, with an intense gaze and a furrowed brow, returned in the center of the gold circle.

"Dawn, who doesn't the child trust—you or me?"

Both of you.

Then again she turned and ran out of the circle. I tried to get her back, but this time I couldn't. The gold ring and the child had disappeared. I told Anne what had happened and she suggested that I open my eyes and again become aware of her office.

When I opened my eyes I felt dazed but completely aware of what had occurred. I focused on Anne. She was watching me closely.

"Anne, why does this child feel she doesn't have a mother? I had a mother."

"I don't know. I think she could tell us a lot about your feelings, but first she's going to have to trust you."

"How do I gain her trust?"

"Stay with her. Make a point of checking in with her at least once a day. Either close your eyes and talk to her, or give her a voice by writing down a question and having her answer it."

"Wouldn't I be imagining her answers?"

"No, not really. That child is very much a part of you. You would be surprised what you can learn about yourself when you give your thoughts and emotions a voice."

I left Anne's office more depressed than when I entered. I drove home in a daze, put the kids down for a nap, then walked into my bedroom closet—my mind was blank, my body was on auto-pilot. I knelt down on the floor, moved some old navy blue pumps out of the corner and curled up against the edge of the wall. A red wool blazer hung over my face, blocking out the dull light of day. Closing my eyes, I wondered why I was in the closet, and why it felt safe, and why I didn't want to leave.

That week, I was a zombie around the house. I'd take a bit of ice cream and put the carton in the refrigerator instead of the freezer. I'd feel a rush of panic when I couldn't remember the day of the week. Thoughts jetted in and out of my head, but nothing seemed to stick. To read a book to my children took all the energy I could muster.

During those days, my friends became a needed blessing. There was six of us moms who helped each other out. We all have children the same age who played together often and as they watch my health decline they spent more time with my children, giving them the love and attention I didn't always have the energy to give. Philip helped as well. He was usually home by three in the afternoon to play with the children and when he was at work, the live-in housekeeper, Malagro, took care of them as if they were her own. I did what I could with the children to nurture them, wishing I had the energy to do more, knowing I would never get back this time in their life. But I wasn't much more alert than a mother going through heavy chemotherapy. Most of the time, I felt like I was on death row with a hangover. And the only relief I experienced was a brief encounter I began to have at night.

After I put the kids to bed one evening, I told Philip I wasn't feeling well and was going to sleep in the other room. I walked into the nest and laid down on the day bed. As my eyes closed and my thoughts floated away, I felt a warm current of air that cocooned my body in a thick, surreal comfort. It felt like a full-bodied woman, a spirit of sort that had the earthy smell of wet red-clay and the deep passion of a rolling sea. Her presence felt strong, enduring, with the substance and beauty of a Indian matron — the wisdom of a spiritual mentor. That night, I fell asleep in her presence. In the morning, I awoke into more pain.

Desperate to find some kind of fast track out of hell, I increased my appointments with Anne to twice, sometimes three times a week.

"Anne, what could possibly be causing so much suffering?" I said as I tossed my keys on the table and flung myself onto the couch. "I feel so isolated, lonely, like I'm a orphan in a prison camp and those feelings just don't coincide with my life."

She stared at me, her eyes touching me like a gentle hand.

"I get worse every day and I'm starting to do strange things."

"What kind of strange things?"

I told her I kept going into the corner of my closet and curling up in a ball.

"That's not that strange. What do you think about when you're in the closet?"

"That I want to die."

She took a deep breath. "Are you suicidal?"

"Wanting to die, and wanting to kill myself are separate feelings. But sometimes I think it's the only way to end my fears and get relief from this pain."

"What keeps you from hurting yourself?"

"Mostly the kids. But there's also a feeling I have. This energy surging through my body keeps telling me there's a reason for all this." Anne looked intrigued, so I went out on a limb and told her about the presence of the woman, the gentle spirit who surrounded me just before I fell asleep.

"Do you communicate with her?"

"In a way, but the communication comes in thoughts, not words. And last night I had the sensation that she was asking permission to work with me, and when I approved I felt a subtle vibration in my body. It's as if the marrow of my bones began to vibrate."

"Is it painful?"

"No, it's soothing, but exhausting. Do you think I'm having a nervous breakdown?"

"No, I think you're going through an psycho-spiritual shift in your body. A metamorphosis."

"A metamorphosis. What am I changing into?"

She smiled. "I don't know, but as long as it's not hurting you, I encourage you to stay with it, and if you can, ask the woman for more information."

"Anne, I think this is all very strange, yet you make it sound almost normal."

"I don't know what the definition of normal is, but I've had similar experiences."

"You have?"

"Yes. I believe changes in our mind affect the chemistry in our bodies."

"But what about the presence?"

"I think you're getting some spiritual guidance to help you through the metamorphosis."

Anne was as comfortable with herself as I had ever seen. Her words soothed me and I wanted to know more.

"Are you religious?" I asked.

She hesitated for a moment, but her shoulders remained relaxed, and her large, blue eyes connecting with mine, soft and inviting. "Let me first ask you that question."

I told her my search for religion had started, and for the most part ended, when I was in junior high — when my friend, Joyce, died in a car accident, in a car I'd almost gotten into. After three days of lying in bed trying to make sense out of her death — and my life — I hopped on my bike and rode to a church on the top of the hill.

"Excuse me, sir…" I said to the priest as I took off my baseball hat and sat across from him in the chapel.

"Call me Father."

"Excuse me, Father, but I was wondering if I could ask you a few questions."

"Certainly. Are you a member of the church?"

"My mom took me to Sunday school once, but I don't really remember it."

"I see. So what brings you here today?"

"I was wondering if you knew what happens when somebody dies?"

He straightened his glasses. "I would have to say that depends on how they lived."

"What do you mean?"

"If they led a good life or if they led a life of sin."

"You mean like lying, cheating, stealing and murder? Sins like that?"

"Yes, those are a few of them, but there are other sins as well. One should not indulge in impure thoughts, engage in sexual activities before marriage, and it's very important that everybody be baptized from original sin."

"Original sin?"

"Yes, you do know about Adam and Eve, don't you?"

"Oh, yes." Although I wasn't sure what the sin was. "Father, if a person follows all the rules, will they go to heaven?"

"According to the Scriptures, they will."

I thought for a moment. "What if you committed a sin, but you didn't know it was a sin?"

"You go to church and pray for God's forgiveness."

"Okay...what if you knew the rules but you sinned anyway?"

"You go to church and pray for God's forgiveness."

I mentally started a list of my transgressions, trying to figure out how much praying I had in store.

"Now is a good time to be considering a church," he said. "Many feel the Judgment Day will come soon."

"What's a Judgment Day?"

"Judgment Day is the end of the world. The day God descends from the heavens and determines if we are worthy to enter His kingdom."

The end of the world! "You mean Judgment Day could happen at any time?"

"Yes, it could."

I thanked the Father and quickly left the church. My thoughts clicked away as I pedaled home. What if Judgment Day came before I had time to pray for forgiveness? What if the rest of my family got into heaven, but I didn't? What if by chance I got into heaven but somebody I loved didn't? Would it still be heaven? Could I even enjoy it?

I pedaled faster as I flew down the hill. Where would God land? Would old people be judged first or would it be in alphabetical order? I turned the corner and cut across a driveway. What about the people that had already died? Did they get judged on Judgment Day or was life like a game of hot potatoes and whoever was stuck on earth when God descended had to suffer through the agonizing process?

By the time I got home I had begun to obsess over the more pressing question: How on earth was I ever going to be worthy enough to get into heaven? I had already told a million lies. And impure thoughts—the mean ones I had about my brother Mark were enough to make me burn in hell. And no sex before marriage? Why would God say that? I hadn't had sex yet, but despite the priest—and my mother's lectures about how it would ruin my reputation—I wasn't planning on waiting until I got married. And what about my dead friend Joyce? There's no way she could make it past those rules.

The next day I sat home on restriction for leaving the house when I was supposed to be on restriction. I plopped down on the couch to watch television and turned to a news report about the starvation in Africa. Staring at the images of naked children, the black flies crawling over their sunken eyes, I thought of the sin, the *original sin*, and I wondered if anybody knew these children needed to be baptized.

I got up the following morning and rode to a different church, my stomach still feeling sick from my encounter with the priest.

"I don't understand," I told the minister. "If God is so good, why do children die? And when they do die, why should they go to hell just because they weren't baptized? They were just kids. They didn't know the rules."

"Dawn," the minister said, "you don't have to worry about the Africans. God exempts children from the rule of baptism." There was a rule of exemption? This was getting confusing. "And I don't think you should be concerned with impure thoughts. Just make sure you catch them before they turn into deeds."

Although sex before marriage was still out, he did present me with a more reasonable belief. Hopeful that I might have found a place of inspiration, I introduced myself to one of the church members, an older woman, who after hearing my concerns, told me, "The only way to heaven is to follow the Lord, our savior Jesus Christ." She emphasized that firm belief in Jesus was the only way into the Kingdom of Heaven.

I walked out of the church more bewildered than when I walked in. Was there really only one way to enter the Kingdom of Heaven? And if there was, why were there so many religions in the world? I didn't know much about God, but it didn't sound right that He would pick one religion and make everybody else wrong.

"I've been to a few Christian churches as an adult," I told Anne, "but some of the interpretations of the Bible still don't make much sense to me."

Anne sympathized with my confusion and shared that she had had her own struggles with her Catholic upbringing.

"Dawn, I think it would help if you understood the difference between spirituality and religion. Spirituality is a part of your being, the relationship you have with your soul. Religion is a belief system that one subscribes to, either in part or in whole."

"Do you belong to a religion?"

"I have my belief system."

"Do you believe in God?"

"Yes, but what God is, and what it means to you, is something you need to discover for yourself."

I felt a deep sense of relief. Finally somebody was telling me something that made sense — something that I could believe.

"So, how do I develop spirituality?"

"You're doing that right now. A psychological healing is a spiritual healing. It's an attempt to bridge the split between your emotional, physical, mental, and spiritual selves. Right now we are getting through the early stages of breaking through some of your barriers — the walls that keep you locked inside a small room instead of enjoying the reality that we all live in a very large house."

"So what do I do next?"

"We keep working with the five-year-old. Have you stayed in contact with her?"

I told Anne that I checked in with her once or twice a day. "Usually after the kids go down for their afternoon naps, I lie face up on the daybed in the nest and close my eyes. I take a few deep breaths and in my mind ask to see the child. A few moments later an image appears of her and me sitting on the white cement curb across the street from the house where I grew up. She's still wearing the same black turtleneck but she doesn't look so leery. She sits close to me but doesn't say much, and then I ask her if she wants a hug, and she crawls into my arms, clinging tightly to me until I open my eyes and come out of the imagery exercise."

"Good, that's exactly what you're supposed to do." Anne said. "Hold that little girl as often as you can. She needs your love right now as much as your children at home do."

"Okay, but I'm still confused about why she's looking for a mother."

"That's all right. I'm sure when she trusts you she'll let you know."

I looked over Anne's shoulder to the clock on the window sill. Our hour was almost over and I wanted to close the session before she did. I stood up and picked up my keys. Anne confirmed our next appointment and opened her arms, as if she was ready to accept every part of me. I smiled and walked into her embrace and as she pulled me in snug against the warmth of her soft body, instead of holding my breath until I pulled away, I stayed in her arms and let go of the breath I had been holding forever.

My sessions with Anne continued and so did my frustrations. Desperate needs for love, affection and security that I deemed weak, offensive and burdensome to others were now all I seemed to be. Ashamed of how much I was beginning to need her, afraid that she wouldn't want to see me if she knew, I began to cover up my desperation with a veil of rational insights and self-promoting behavior.

I boasted about a political career that I now felt was my destiny — a high ranking position where I could channel the energy I felt barreling through my body. Anne appeared to enjoy my enthusiasm, while I waited — even hoped — for her to call me on my arrogance.

When I left her office I'd come home, my body leading me back into the corner of my bedroom closet. With her perfume still lingering on my sweater, I'd curl up in a ball, wishing I had the nerve to tell her that what I really needed was for her to take me home, hold me in her arms and give me a safe place to cry. A place that wouldn't end in an hour. A place where I could trust her to care for me because she wanted to, not because I paid her for it.

I didn't think I could get that kind of relationship from therapy, and I still wasn't sure why I wanted it, so I kept my desires to myself and tested her relentlessly. How quickly would she call me back if I left a message? How flexible would she be in making my appointments? And if I was going to continue to get involved in our relationship, how involved was she willing to become?

I entered our next session looking for some security, trying to cover up my need for it.

"Anne, you know how you said I'm going to need to trust you?"

"It would help."

"If I trust you to care for me, I would like to know you have something at stake."

She looked puzzled. "Help me understand what you need."

"I'm really not interested in going to the depths of my soul while you sit behind some wall of authority and take notes about it. If I'm going to have an emotional investment in this relationship, I want you to have one too."

"I already do."

"You do?"

"Yes. I do." She said it like she meant it. She said it like she was trying to tell me that she loved me. "But," her voice began to harden, "there are therapeutic guidelines, boundaries I need to set for your protection."

"My protection? I can take care of myself."

"I don't think you understand the dynamics involved in therapy. You could become very vulnerable here, even dependent."

Dependent. I couldn't stand to hear the word.

"I'm not going to get dependent. I've never needed anyone, and I have no intention of starting."

"For a while, you might need to depend on me. You might need to trust that I can support you while you let go of the strong hold you have on yourself. I want you to know that it is all right to let me care for you."

I shook my head. "No, it isn't. Anne, you have a life outside of this office. A life that could take you out of here at any time."

"You're right, I do have a life. But part of my life is my job, and right now that job is to take care of you and help you through this depression."

"Why do you care if I get through it?"

"Because you're worth caring for, and I fully intend to do so for as long as you need me. You can trust me, Dawn, I'm not going anywhere."

I wanted to believe her, but I didn't.

"I don't need anybody to take care of me, I just need to be understood. Ever since I was a little kid, I fantasized about having somebody come into my life and see right through me—see how scared I've been and give me the love, acceptance, and understanding that I need."

"We all want that."

"We do?"

"Sure. I think there is a deep yearning for wholeness and understanding in every human being, but I don't think you're going to find it from somebody else."

I rolled my eyes.

"Dawn, I believe that's what that child is trying to tell you. You need to find your own self-love and compassion. And when you learn how to love, accept and understand yourself, you will be able to share in that with others."

"Anne, I don't believe in that bullshit that I'm my own hero. I've spent my whole life being there for me, and I'll tell you, it's lonely and unfulfilling."

"I think if you really look at your life you might find that you have been protecting yourself from your thoughts, not trying to understand where they came from or who you really are. You may think it's bullshit, but we can only receive love to the extent that we can love ourselves."

"Well, that might be how it is, but it still feels like if the right person knew how to love me the pain would finally go away."

"Dawn, I'll give you what I can, but you need to remember something very important about our relationship."

"What's that?"

"The hunger and yearning you feel to be held, and to be loved, is from the child inside of you who wants a mother. That mother needs to be you. I can't fill that role."

I looked at the floor. A stab of rejection was piercing through my stomach. It was taking everything I had to cover the pain.

"I know this might sound harsh," she said, "but I'm not here to feed you. I'm here to teach you how to fish."

"Then I'll try to learn quickly, because right now I'm starving to death."

Chapter 3

I sat in the nest at night imaging the child. She was a five-year-old sitting on the asphalt curb, her nose peeling from sunburn, her feet leathery from refusing to wear shoes. I'd ask the child questions she wouldn't answer, then I'd take her in my arms and her mind would become mine. I was a little girl trapped in a pitch-black alley, my back against the wall, my breathing so shallow it had almost stopped. Killers lurked around me listening for my voice; my silence and the darkness were my only protection.

As the days continued to shorten, I found myself more often in the closet. The corners of the walls seemed to hold my own structure intact, giving me a sense of security while my thoughts unraveled into babbling phrases.

"They're going to kill me!"

Who was going to kill me? Who? My heart began to race and my body broke out in a cold sweat.

I opened my eyes and phoned Anne. I arranged to meet her the following day.

Anne embraced me as soon as I walked into her office.

"Are you okay?"

"This feels so crazy."

"Do you remember anything or anyone who could have threatened your life?"

"I've been thinking about it all night. The only thing I can remember is a man who once tried to lure me into his car."

Anne looked alarmed. "Why didn't you tell me this before?"

"It was nothing. I was riding out in front of my house on my scooter and this man stopped at the street corner and asked me for directions. By the time I got within a hundred feet of his car, I knew the guy was a kidnapper and I turned around and ran."

"How did you know he was a kidnapper?"

"I could tell by the way he was staring at me. He was sitting in his idling blue sedan, looking at me as if I was an animal he wanted to eat for dinner."

"Where did you run to?"

"I rode my scooter back to the house, grabbed my brother and sister off the front lawn and pulled them into the house."

"Do you remember anything else? Anything that happened after you ran in the house?"

"I remember locking the doors and closing the curtains. My mom kept asking me what I was doing. I didn't want to tell her because I thought it would scare her, so I just kept yelling at her to not let the kids go outside."

"Wait a minute. You didn't want to scare your mom? What about your fear?"

"I thought she'd overreact if she knew somebody had tried to kidnap me and that would have made the whole thing worse."

"Did you ever tell her?"

"Yes, a few hours later I did — when I was calm and I knew the danger was gone."

"Did anybody call the police?"

"Probably not. Anne, do you think this is what has me so scared?"

"I'm not sure, but if you don't mind I'd like to do a guided imagery on the memory to see if we can get some more details."

I was afraid to close my eyes, then I looked into Anne's face. It was clear she wasn't going to let anything bad happen to me.

I closed my eyes and sat back in the chair. Comforted by the music in the background and the light, smoky-sweet smell of her perfume in the air, I took a few breaths and listened to her suggestions. Her voice was soft and deep.

"When you're ready, I want you to go back to the day you were five years old and the man stopped in front of your house."

The image of his car came up immediately. "He's driving an old blue sedan with a big dent on the door. I'm riding in the street on my red scooter when he stops."

"What happens next?"

"He stares at me for a while, then he asks my name. He tells me he has something for me. I need to come into his car to see it."

"What happens next?"

"I can't move. My whole body feels locked up. He asks me again to come up to his car and I bolt on my scooter toward the house. I pull my little brother off his tricycle and then pick up my sister off the lawn. She's so little, I'm afraid he's going to get her."

"You're okay, just stay with it and tell me what happens next."

"I'm in the house locking the doors. I'm angry and scared, and there's nobody here to help me." My voice started to crack. Every muscle in my body was tense.

"Is your mother there?"

"Yes... but... but you don't understand. There's nobody here... there's nobody here to help me!"

"Go get your mother or father. Bring in an adult who can help you."

A distant image of my parents came into my mind — my mother kneeling on the living room carpet, the dark shadow of my father standing behind her. I felt a panic rising in my chest and I lost control of my thoughts. "No. No. No! I don't want to know this! I don't want to know this! I'll die if I know this!"

My body broke into a tremor of terror. My legs bouncing with the desire to run for my life. I opened my eyes and jumped to my feet.

"I don't want to know this, Anne. I really don't want to know this."

"Dawn, it's okay, you're safe. You need to keep telling yourself that. You are safe."

"No, I'm not! This is death. Something is going to kill me." I brought my knees to my chest and covered my head with my hands, as terrified as if a mad man had a gun to my head.

"Dawn. I want you to breathe and to look at me." Her voice sounded calm, but urgent.

I looked into the light in her eyes. There I saw safety; I saw love. I felt myself calming down.

"Keep breathing," she said. "Your mind is dealing with something in the past; whatever it is, it has already happened. You need to keep telling yourself that." She leaned forward and the air between us felt warm, safe. I took a deep breath and released the clinch in my jaw. "It has already happened and you're safe now."

"Why am I so scared?

"I don't know. I'm as confused about this as you are."

"Do you think I was abused by somebody?"

"There's no way of telling. It could have been a lot of things. You might have almost drowned in the tub when no one was looking. You could have been trapped someplace and thought you were going to die. There are so many things that a child's mind can perceive as fearful that you can't jump to any conclusions. When you're safe enough with yourself to understand what happened to you, your mind will let you know."

I ran my palms down the front of my jeans trying to dry the sweat off my hands. "Anne, I've been depressed for almost a year. I don't know how much more of this I can stand."

She looked at me as if she wanted to come over and hold me. "It's times like these I wish I did have a quick fix for this process. I know this work is difficult, but I promise you it will not last forever."

My hour was up and I had no place to go. I picked up my keys and stared at her, hoping she wouldn't make me leave.

"Rub your feet against the floor and breathe."

We looked at each other for the next few minutes and when my eyes cleared up she came over and hugged me.

"Dawn, I have faith in you. This is all going to make sense someday. I know it will."

I went home and called my mom to ask if I had ever had a near drowning experience or anything similar that would make me feel I was going to die. There was nothing out of the ordinary that she could remember.

"We did the best we could with you," she said.

"I'm not blaming you for anything. I'm just looking for some information."

"Dawn, it was always hard to tell whether anything ever happened to you. When you were scared or hurt, you just got angry and pushed everybody away — and you did that a lot."

She was right; if something ever had happened to me, I wouldn't have gone to anyone for help. Least of all her. I hung up the phone and walked down to the kitchen, ashamed to think of what she was telling my father. She'd make light of my suffering, act as though I was on a tangent. He'd be lying on the couch listening, chuckling, thinking I had too much time on my hands, too much money in my pockets.

I picked up the kids from pre-school, ran some errands to keep them entertained, then came home and put in a video. When Phil came home, I went to bed, sleeping through dinner and falling into a dream. In the dream, my father paced in front of me while I sat motionless in an old, tan leather chair.

"You've gone far enough," he said as he shook his finger at me. "I want you to stop this ridiculous therapy and get back to work. Do you hear me? Get back to work!"

I felt a familiar humiliation as I sank deep into the chair.

"Do you hear me?" he said. "Stop now. Don't go any further."

In our next session, I told Anne about my nightmare.

"Do you think it means anything?" I said.

"I don't know. Do you think your father disapproves of therapy?"

"Disapproves is probably not the right word. I think he doesn't believe in it. My dad thinks people should just work hard and appreciate what they have."

"So he doesn't see therapy as a way to gain knowledge?"

"No. I think he thinks it's a way of creating problems that don't exist."

"What do you think?"

"I think people can over-analyze their problems, but I don't think that's what we're doing."

"No. I don't either. I think something very real has scared that five-year-old child."

I looked at her, feeling as if she knew me in a way nobody had ever known me.

"How is the child doing?" she said.

"She's scared."

"We could try another guided imagery if you're up to it."

"I'm not, but I don't see where I have a choice anymore."

She smiled. "You always have a choice."

"Between what, hell or hell?"

"I'm sorry it feels that way."

Her compassion briefly lightened the heaviness in my body. I leaned back in my chair and closed my eyes.

"Take a few deep breaths," she said, "and let go of all the thoughts of the day. When you're ready, I want you to go back to your five-year-old body. Back to the day the man asked you into his car."

I remembered grabbing my brother and sister off the lawn and running inside the house. My bedroom window faced the street and

I tried to go there first to close the curtains. But when I entered the hall to my bedroom my feet pushed me back onto Anne's couch.

"I'm afraid! I want to stop now!"

"Take a few deep breaths and try to stay with the image. Bring your mom or dad in to help you."

I was panting, the words coming straight from my chest. "I'm not safe here, I'm not safe... I have to protect myself."

"Dawn, I want you to keep breathing and go to a place where you felt safe. There must have been some place in your life where you knew you were safe. I want you to go there now and tell me where you are."

I felt slightly dizzy. It was difficult to stay conscious as the image of a large-framed woman sitting with her legs crossed appeared in the inside of my mind. It felt like the same spirit I had been feeling at night. An Indian matron with creamy, dark skin and large, brown eyes that appeared slightly oriental. She had a tranquil beauty. Her long, thick, black hair was loosely tied back and fell to the side of the soft orange shawl wrapped around her shoulders. In her arms, held tightly against her breast by long dark fingers, was the form of a healthy round infant. Below the Indian woman was an image of my mother lying on a bed with the extended girth of a woman in her last trimester.

I explained the image to Anne and as I did, my consciousness merged with the child in the Indian matron's arms. My hands, feet, and chest began to warm. My heart felt as thought it was opening as I entered an all-encompassing state of peace.

"What's happening to you?" Anne said.

"I'm safe here. Wherever I am, I'm safe." A moment later, the image disappeared and I slowly opened my eyes.

Anne stared at me. "You're glowing. You look like you could light up the entire city."

"This place in my mind, it's like heaven."

My eyes came into focus and I looked at Anne. There was a glow around her, a love in her eyes that looked like the love I was in.

"I feel healed," I said. "Like I've been forgiven."

"Maybe you have."

Our session was almost over. I thanked Anne with a long embrace, our bodies fitting together so snugly it felt as if we were one. Then I peacefully floated out of the room.

When I pulled up in the driveway, Philip was standing in the garage. His tall, broad-shouldered frame, sandy-brown hair and sky blue eyes were as beautiful as I had ever seen. I walked up and gave him a kiss. He stared at me as though we hadn't met.

"You look like the happiest person I've ever seen," he said.

I described the experience I'd had in the session, and we both held on to the hope that the feeling would be permanent.

The following afternoon I went up to the nest to take a nap. When I closed my eyes I saw an image of myself falling backwards from the sky. The love, peace and wholeness that had filled me was gone. The grieving had returned, along with a headache that felt like a slight hangover.

In my next session, Anne and I talked about the heightened experience. She could see my serenity had worn off and asked what caused the change.

"I think my thoughts did," I said. "I went from feeling completely whole and loved, to the feeling like I was falling from heaven. The guilt and remorse poured back into my chest and stomach, as if I'd recalled doing something shamefully wrong. Those beliefs have so much power over me, thinking of them pulled me right back into my suffering."

"How do you feel now?"

"I feel the same heavy pain I felt before I experience the wholeness and serenity, but now I know there's hope."

"It's so good to hear you say that. Dawn, where did you go to feel so safe and at peace?"

"I became an pre-borne infant in the arms of an Indian spirit. A woman who, in some way, felt connected to me."

"What else did you notice about the woman?"

"She felt like the same presence or spirit I feel in my room at night. The one I feel right before I fall asleep." I stared through the window, recalling the image. "She looks like an oil painting I have over my fireplace. A portrait of an Indian woman, sitting with her legs crossed against a misty, light-gray backdrop." I pulled up my arms and showed Anne how the woman's hands came up from under her shawl, positioned as if she was holding an infant. "Although there isn't a baby in the portrait, she is looking into her arms with the compassion and tranquility of a mother late at night nursing her newborn."

The air around Anne and me felt magical. Our eyes stayed connected while Anne asked how I acquired the picture. I told her about a trip Phil and I had taken to Palm Springs. Samantha was still in diapers and the three of us were wandering through an art show. The oil painting of the Indian woman was displayed on an aisle along with several other paintings by an artist name Franco. I was telling Phil how much the painting moved me when the artist came up and asked our names.

"This painting needs to be with you," he said in a strong Italian accent.

I laughed at his salesmanship. "I love your work, but we just purchased a house and are a little low on funds."

The artist turned to Phil and asked how much he had. Phil offered him a few hundreds dollars which was a fraction of the price.

The artist took a long look at Samantha, her bright blue eyes always reflecting a wisdom way beyond her years. "I'll take it," the artist said to Phil.

While Phil paid the clerk, the artist ran over to get another painting of the same woman. In this portrait, she was seated next to a large Indian pot, looking pensive, her long brown fingers crossed over her half bent knees. "Keep these pictures together," he said, "they were meant to be with you." He smiled brightly and handed the second one to me. I returned the smile, warmed by the sight of the painting and his generosity.

Anne continued to light up. "This is only my opinion," she said, "but I don't think you got the image of the woman because of the picture. I tend to agree with the artist. The pictures needed to be with you."

It was one of those rare days I left therapy feeling better than when I walked in. The grieving was debilitating, but through its darkness I knew I was incubating something new. And I knew it was leading me to something beyond my pain and suffering.

I awoke the next morning in the nest. The sun was shining through the steam on the glass window, and I wiped it away to reveal a crisp, blue horizon. I got up before Phil and the kids and walked to the beach. The brisk winter day invigorated my senses, and I picked up my pace and ran to the sand.

At the end of the shoreline, I climbed up on a bluff and sat down to watch the ocean. Beneath me, I heard the water swelling against the cliff. Above me a seagull called for its mate. I took a deep breath of the clear salt air and canvassed the face of the ocean. The calm blue water looked solid in mass, the subtle rhythm of the tide the only sign of motion. I followed the current with my eyes and began to feel a soft, soothing elation. When my awareness came back to myself, the spirit of the Indian woman was with me. Her dense and peaceful aura surrounded my body and a message entered my mind.

Love yourself.

"Love myself?" I said it out loud and her presence disappeared. I thought I did love myself, even though I wasn't sure I knew what love was.

I climbed down from the bluff and walked up the beach. The peace of the encounter was still with me, and so was the notion that loving myself was not just an idea, it was a requirement.

That night I was putting the kids to bed. Halfway through *The Cat In The Hat*, I realized that Michael and Erica were asleep in my arms. I carried them to bed, then curled up with Samantha. The nightlight cast a soft glow on her long, dark eyelashes, freckled, round face and thick, straight, blonde hair. Her two front teeth had fallen out and her legs now reached all the way down to my knees. She was such a special joy to me. A gift beyond anything I could have ever dreamed.

"Samantha..."

"Yeah?"

"Do you love yourself?"

"Yeah, Mom, I do."

"How do you know?"

She smiled. "Well, at night, right before I go to sleep, I think about all the people I love, and all of a sudden, I pop up. Sometimes I'm at the beginning of the list, sometimes I'm at the end, and sometimes I just pop up in the middle."

How does she know so much?

"That's really neat."

"Yeah, I even have a name for it." She started to giggle. "I call it the Sammy Whammy."

"The Sammy Whammy." I chuckled. "It sure sounds like you have a lot of love."

"I have so much it feels like I'm going to explode. Sometimes at school I just have to get rid of it, so I run up to my teacher and give her a great big hug." Her eyes twinkled. "But, the funny thing is, when you try to give love away, it comes right back at ya."

"I bet your teacher loves having you in her class."

"Mom, I think she loves everybody."

I smiled. Samantha's first grade teacher was the kind of woman who did seem to love everybody.

We kissed goodnight. "You'd better get some sleep now, buddy."

I crawled into my bed and turned off the light. Philip was in the garage playing pool with a friend. I rolled over and hugged my pillow to my chest, then closed my eyes and thought of all the people I loved. Faces and names popped into my head, but my own was nowhere in sight.

I sat in the waiting room to Anne's office. A woman who must have weighed three hundred pounds walked out of a session with another therapist. I smiled at her as she passed. A year ago, I wouldn't have acknowledged her, would have condemned her for what seemed to me a lack of self control. Today I wondered what it would be like to be her.

"Dawn, come on back." I looked up from my chair and saw Anne. When our eyes met I felt my breathe catch, and as a warm smile came to my face, I realized my infatuation with her was growing.

"Okay," I said once we where in her office. "Let's try again."

"Are you sure that's what you want to do?"

"Yes, I'm sure."

"You're a courageous woman."

"Actually, I'm just too scared to stay still." The fear that I was about to die now gripped every fiber of my body.

"Okay, when you're ready, close your eyes." She gave me several suggestions to relax, then asked me again to remember myself as a five-year-old.

When I closed my eyes I saw black, then I allowed my mind to float off and a few moments later I began to see images inside my head.

"This is strange," I said.

"What's that?"

"I see myself as a Chinese girl. I'm wandering through a rice field. The grass around me is taller than I am...the water almost comes up to my knees."

"How do you know it's you?" she said.

"I see her, but I am her. I know what she's thinking and feeling."

"How old are you?"

"Five. I'm scared that I can't find my mother." My chest tightened and I started to pant.

"Look around. Tell me what you see."

I came across an old Asian woman, lying face up in the shallow water with one arm limp around her head.

"I found my grandmother. She's dead in the field."

"What do you want to do?"

"I want to find my mom." I was on the verge of tears.

"Then keep looking."

I ran through the fields searching in the grass, then noticed a pressure building in my chest. My breathing became labored. My chest felt like it was about to collapse. I saw the image of the hoof of a horse and a wooden stick with a dragon carved in the handle. I was about to lose consciousness from the pressure on my chest when white light rushed in, threatening to absorb me.

My eyes flew open and I jumped to my feet. "What the hell was that?"

"I don't know," Anne said. "You're the one taking me on this journey. Tell me what's happening to you."

I paced across the floor. "I don't know. It was like a memory... but the feelings are current. I'm still looking for my mother."

I sat down again and looked over at Anne. "What do you think that was about?"

"I can't say for sure. How do you feel?"

"My chest feels lighter, but my mind's boggled."

Anne spent the rest of the session teaching me ways to ground my awareness. She showed me how to do a meditation to root my feet in the earth, to help me be more present in my thoughts and more comfortable with unusual images.

"Why don't you go home and write about what you experienced today," she said as we finished. "I'll call you in the morning to see how you're doing."

I left the session confused. The experience was not like a dream, because I was conscious the entire time. I thought for a moment that the images might have been part of a television show or movie I'd seen. But that didn't explain the intense physical symptoms I felt when the horse crushed me, or the relief in my chest when the memory was over. Although I didn't believe in reincarnation, a past-life experience was the only explanation that made any sense.

I came home and told Phil what had happened.

"You must have been in the era of the Ming Dynasty," he said. "The Chinese rulers used to conquer the land by sending in troops of soldiers who rode through the fields and crushed the citizens and farm workers."

"You mean you believe in reincarnation?"

"I never used to, but do you remember a few years ago when we went down to the Mayan ruins?"

"Yes."

"When we entered Tulum, I had the strangest experience. The sights and smells all began to change. The tourists disappeared, and I saw myself as a Mayan in a working community."

"Did you think it was just your imagination?"

"No, it was much different than a fantasy or a dream. It was like I was stuck in a dèjá vu for several minutes. I didn't tell you about it because I didn't think you would understand, but it felt like I once lived there."

I felt my mind opening from the absurdity. "We better not tell anybody about this," I said. "I think you can get thrown out of the Republican party from talking about past life experiences."

That night I called Anne and told her that I thought my experience in the guided imagery session my have been a past-life memory. But I was still skeptical about the concept.

"I've seen many clients spontaneously enter what appear to be past-life experiences," she said. She emphasized that it was not important to believe in reincarnation for the experience to release and heal both emotional and physical pain.

"Anne, do you think what's frightening me happened in a past life?"

"It could have."

"Do you believe in past lives?"

"Yes, I do. I've seen too much evidence not to."

It was a depressing turn in my therapy. Digging up the past thirty years was hard enough; the thought of my pain being rooted in a past life made me feel I was opening up an endless can of worms.

I spent the next week in the library trying to find some evidence that would help make my experience more understandable. I read countless published accounts of psychiatrists, psychologists and medical doctors who reported findings similar to what I had experienced. Several sources said that through regression therapy, people commonly re-experienced what appears to be a traumatic past-life death. It is also common for that memory to release repressed emotions and heal the wounds that had manifested in the behavior, or in the physical body of a current life.

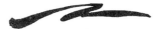

Anne and I spent the next few sessions talking about my experiences in guided imagery, and my deepening depression. I needed some time to digest the surge of new information, and I was also becoming concerned about my growing dependency on her. My silent struggle between pride and insecurity continued to rage in my head. More than ever I needed to trust that she cared for me, but her skillful techniques to maintain our therapeutic relationship, and her genuine personal feelings for me were becoming harder and harder to distinguish.

"Are you sure you're ready for another guided imagery session?" Anne asked in our next session.

"Like you said, whatever it is, it already happened."

"Okay, then, when you're ready, close your eyes and take a few deep breaths."

The piano solo playing from a small stereo box on the floor of Anne's office soothed me into the flooding sensation. Anne asked me to let go of my thoughts with every breath.

"When you're ready, I want you to go back to the front of your childhood home."

I began to focus on my surroundings.

"Where are you?" she said.

With my eyes closed, I looked down and saw myself as an older man in a brown-hooded robe.

"I'm in a monastery. I'm sitting in a large wooden chair in a room next to the front entrance." Guilt and fear surged through my body. "There's an army outside the door. They've come to kill me."

"Why do they want to kill you?"

"I have taken their soldiers into my church." The feelings of remorse for my behavior was unbearable. "I have persuaded these young men to come into the sanctuary and then I used them as servants and slaves. Oh God, I should never have done that."

"Stay with the feelings and tell me what happens next."

"My hands are tied behind me and bound to a tall wooden pole staked into the ground several yards from the front of my church. The men circle around the pole and start a fire beneath me. I feel terrible for what I've done. I have sinned and I deserve to be punished."

The flames rose to my eyes and I felt myself leaving that body, rising above the heat, feeling as if a war that had threatened me for years was finally over.

"Dawn, why are you remembering this lifetime? Is there anything significant you need to learn?"

Her question brought up the image of the Indian woman. Far in the background, I saw a small bright light that looked like a distant star. There were other images around the light, but I couldn't make out what they were.

"The Indian woman is here... and a light that looks very far away." I opened my eyes for a moment and looked around the room for an overhead lamp that might be causing the image, but the room was dim with diffused light. I closed my eyes again and a few moments later the image re-appeared.

"This is really strange, but there's a light in my head."

"What does the light want?"

"It wants to talk to me...it wants me to come closer. Anne, this is scaring me. I don't want to go near the light."

"It's all right. You can stay right where you are. Does the Indian woman scare you?"

"No."

"Okay, the life as a monk that you just recalled — ask the woman why you remembered it. What was the lesson or meaning in that life?"

The image of the Indian woman, crossing her legs in a seated position stayed constant as telepathic thoughts entered my mind. As I heard myself repeat them, I began to understand the significance.

"Honesty. I must never misuse my power or mislead other people."

"If you agree to do that, can you let go of your guilt?"

"Not yet. There is still more to learn."

Anne paused. "Before you leave this image, I want you to ask the Indian woman what lesson you are working on in this life."

"*Trust.*"

I opened my eyes and brought my consciousness back to the room. Anne and I talked about the messages. She explained that the images and information I was receiving were not abnormal for the type of work we were doing. "That's why I prefer to work with guided imagery," she said. "The information is very insightful and it's coming from you. You are always going to know what you need to encounter and when."

"You mean the Indian woman is a part of me?"

"Yes. I think spiritual guides represent a deeper, wiser part of the mind."

"What about the lessons?" I asked. "What's that all about?"

"What do you think?"

"I think I came into this world with more on my mind than a blank slate."

"It does appear that way. You look a little dazed. How do you feel?"

I thought for a moment. "Sad. Alone. I hurt all the time, and I still don't know why."

Anne's eyes looked as sad as I felt. "I know this is hard work," she said, "but your pain is productive. We often can't see where we're going in the darkness, but I promise, you are making progress."

"My heart feels so congested. For once in my life I just wish I could cry."

She looked at the clock. "Next session," she said, "I want you to wear comfortable clothes and bring a blanket or pillow—anything you can hold that will help you feel more secure. I'll block off extra time for you and we'll try another guided imagery session to get some relief. I want those tears for you as much as you do."

"That sounds good."

She stood up and opened her arms. I walked into them like a child who had found a safe home, and she held me, as if she had been waiting to love me for a very long time.

At night the vibrations in my body continued, along with an occasional encounter with the Indian woman. The night after my session with Anne, the spirit of the woman re-appeared. I was at my desk writing notes in a calendar when the surrealistic sensation of her presence sedated me. Her energy felt natural, the way it felt to be lying on a warm rock, next to a clear stream in the middle of an enchanting forest. I closed my eyes.

It's time you knew the truth about your father.

I opened my eyes and wrote down the message. Time I know the truth about my father? What did that mean?

Anne called and canceled our next appointment. She had plans to visit a friend in San Francisco and had forgotten to mention it in our last session. I acted unaffected and hung up the phone. *I'll block out extra time for you. Bring something to feel secure. I want those tears for you as much as you do.* How the hell through all of that could she forget to tell me she wasn't going to be there?

My chest had begun its meltdown. Suddenly feeling as if I were a child and my mother had just left me destitute. I floored myself in the nest for the rest of the evening, confused by how much her cancellation hurt me, loathing myself for how weak I'd become.

I walked into our next session and tossed down my keys.

"How was your trip?" I said.

"Fine. We had a good time."

"Good. Will you give me your home phone number?"

"That came out of left field. Why do you want it?"

"I want to know you trust me enough to have your home phone number."

She looked perplexed. "Why is this coming up right now?"

"Mainly because I hate being in this position, and if I get in a place where I need immediate help, I don't want to talk to your damn recorder."

"That sounds reasonable, but where is the anger coming from?"

"Like I told you. I don't like my downtrodden position here. It's very uncomfortable for me to need you as much as I do and to know that you don't need me at all."

"It's not necessary for me to need you, to care for you."

I wanted to scream. "Anne, I'm living in the bowels of hell right now and, unfortunately, you're my only lifeline. How am I supposed to trust you're not going to drop the rope when you blow off a session that doesn't mean shit to you."

"My vacation." Her eyes grew larger. "Oh, God, I'm so sorry. I didn't mean to cancel with such short notice, but I really thought I had told you about it in our last session."

"No, in our last session we planned to block off extra time so we could try to get me some relief from this pain."

She hung her head as if the stupidity of her own actions was weighing her down.

"Anne, I know I'm just a time slot to you. You can walk away from me without a thought. But I can't. I'm stuck here and, as much as I hate it, I need you."

"Dawn, there are many things that I think about when I think of you. But never have I thought of you as a time slot. I care for you very much and, although I'm human and I make mistakes, my intentions are to be with you until you don't need me. And, believe it or not, someday that will happen. Sooner or later you're going to walk out of this office strong, secure, and no longer in need of me or my services."

I couldn't conceive of a day when I wouldn't want her in my life.

"How can I make this up to you?" she said.

"I don't know. I feel so frustrated here."

"What would make you more comfortable?"

"I guess if I could see you someplace else. Someplace out of here where I could find out who you are."

"We can't leave here; it's against the therapeutic boundaries."

I rolled my eyes. "What are the therapeutic boundaries?"

"There are several, but, generally speaking, the relationship between a therapist and client should stay within the confines of the therapeutic environment. In this case, this would refer to my office."

"Great. I enter this eight-foot room twice a week to bare my soul to you and I don't have any idea who you are. I don't know who you hang out with. What your husband's like. I don't even know where you live. I have no way of gauging you as a person."

"How do you normally gauge people?"

"By their actions and their friendships. How they interact with me in the world, not in a therapeutic box."

"Dawn, you can test me all you want as your therapist, but I can't give you a friendship."

I hate this game. "I'm friends with my accountants. What's the difference?"

"This is a very intimate relationship—it needs to be protected."

"Protected! You're the one being protected here. I can't call you direct, I have to leave a message. You set up our appointments when you have time. Your life is a mystery and mine's an open book. It's all a demeaning reminder that I'm the psycho case here and you're protected from me by your rules."

"They are not my rules, they are the ethics that govern the industry, and they are designed to protect the client, not the therapist. I support them because they are in your best interest."

"If I didn't make the rules, how could they be in my best interest?" I grabbed my keys off the table. "This relationship makes me feel like a child, and I'm not one. I'm a responsible person, and I exercise good judgment, and I want to be respected for that."

She shook her head. "Dawn, I have a great deal of respect for you. I don't understand what's behind this, but within my limitations, I want to do whatever I can to help you."

I stared at her. "I'm a maverick, Anne; I can't be corralled in a small room like this."

"I know this process is difficult for you."

"I'm not sure you do."

Tears welled on the rims of her eyes. "Dawn, I am so sorry that I hurt you."

I felt her pain, but I had nothing to say. I opened the door and walked out.

"Are you coming back?" she said.

"Yeah... I'll be back."

That night I felt great. Anne was hurting, because she knew she hurt me. She cared. And her tearful apology gave me more strength than I'd had in a year. I cranked up some music and rallied the kids. We cleaned out drawers, packed up old clothes, and pulled the dead leaves off the house plants. I knew my energy was at the expense of Anne's remorse, but that didn't seem to bother me until I walked into my room. I was heading toward the nest, bobbing to the B52's, *Love Shack,* when a wave of sorrow grabbed at my chest and dropped me to my knees. I closed my eyes. What was this?

Don't leave her in this pain.

I caught my breath, and a glimpse of the realization. Anne Myers was a part of me—a part of me I didn't know but one I shouldn't hurt. I called Anne and left a message. Ten minutes later she returned my call, the sorrow still heavy in her voice.

"Anne, I'm all right. You don't need to feel bad about this any longer."

There was a pause. "Dawn, I appreciate the call, but you don't need to take care of me."

"If you feel as bad as I do, then taking care of you is taking care of me."

I told her about the sudden feelings I found myself in and how they felt as if they were not mine, but hers. She seemed shocked to admit that the feelings I described were the feelings she was having, and her voice became softer, more intimate.

"I can't tell you how sorry I am. I know the work we are doing together is very important and the last thing I ever, ever wanted to do was add to your pain."

"I know."

"Dawn, I want more than anything to be able to help you, and I know I can't do that unless you trust me."

"I do trust you. I have never experienced someone else's feelings, like I did with you tonight. I don't know what all is going on in this relationship, but after today I trust it, and I trust you."

We said good night with the intimacy of lovers. Not because of the words but because of the intensity behind them. There was something about our relationship, a mystery beyond what either of us could see, and while her job was to keep it within the boundaries, mine was to make sure she didn't negate it.

At the beginning of our next session Anne handed me a piece of paper.

"Here's my home phone number. I live in Dana Point, and my husband's name is Dave."

I was touched by her gesture.

"I want you to know that I trust you very much," she said.

"Thank you. I promise I won't call you unless I have a gun to my head."

"Promise you'll call me before you even consider such a thing."

I smiled. "I promise."

"Are you ready to get down to work?"

"Sure. Where are we going?"

"I want to keep it general this time. Why don't you close your eyes?"

She gave me a few suggestions to relax and then began the guided imagery.

"When you're ready, I want you to go back to the origin of your fears."

I continued to relax for another minute or two and then became aware of the image of the Indian woman.

"The Indian woman's here."

"Okay, ask her if she has anything she wants to tell you today."

It's important to experience past-life images, but you need to stop looking there. Everything you need to know can be found in the present.

I repeated the message to Anne. Then, the image faded and I opened my eyes.

"Do you understand the messages you just received?" Anne said.

"I understand that my thoughts have evolved through time, and are present in my current life. Anne, whatever happened to me, happened in this life. I don't have to time travel anymore." My arms felt to my sides as a layer of weight rose from my chest.

She nodded slowly and pressed on. "If you look at some of the feelings you have found in the inner-child work and the perceptions you have as an adult, you might find a theme in your life. Something that you perceive as continually happening to you."

"I don't know, there's so much here. I often feel somebody wants to kill me and I'm in great danger. There are feelings of abandonment, guilt, and mistrust. The Indian woman gave me a message that it's time I know the truth about my father. And I still have the yearning to be held by a woman. I don't really know where to begin."

"When did you get that message about your father?"

"A couple of weeks ago."

"Did it mean anything to you?"

"No, not really."

She tapped her pencil for a moment, then wrote the word *Love* on a clipboard and handed me the paper.

"I want you to write a sentence using this word."

I scribbled out my first reaction:

Love hurts, it can't be trusted, and it always leaves.

I handed back the clipboard.

"When in your life have you experienced this?"

"Let's see...when my older brother, James, left for college. When my husband, Phil, who was then my boyfriend, left for college. And then a few years later when Phil broke up with me."

"Why did he break up with you?"

I cringed at the memory of my twenty-first birthday. Phil hadn't been very attentive and it seemed he was only taking me to dinner out of a sense of obligation. He probably would have waited until morning to give me the bad news, but I pushed him to find out what was wrong and he finally blurted it out.

"I don't love you any more."

I showed no reaction, but you could have mopped me off the floor like a puddle of toxic waste. I was devastated.

"Ouch," Anne said. "That must have hurt."

"Not as much as it did a week later when I found out he had another girl friend."

Anne winced.

"He came back, but emotionally I never did. The pain almost killed me, and I decided not to risk it again, not even after I married him."

"Can you describe the pain?"

"Abandonment. Betrayal. I had just turned fifteen when my brother left. I remember coming out of the depression with an almost superhuman will to survive without him. I was a rock, a lone island, and I was never going to love anybody again."

"How did Phil get through those walls?"

"I don't know. In fact, I didn't know I loved him until he left for college and I went home and crawled into bed for a week. I figured I must have fallen in love. What else could hurt that bad?"

"So when you wrote down, 'love hurts, it can't be trusted and it always leaves,' that is truly how you experience love?"

"Yes, until I had Samantha."

"How was that different?"

I didn't know how to explain it. My baby girl nursing at my breasts, rooted me to earth like I'd never been rooted before. And the affection that poured out of me, like she'd tapped an unknown geyser straining to be released.

"She needed to be loved," I said. "And it felt safe to love her."

"So you're safe to experience love only if somebody's needs depend on it?"

"I guess."

Anne shook her head. "Dawn, when you get home I want you to start writing with the sentence, 'I felt abandoned when...' and then set a timer for five minutes. Keep your pen moving the entire time, even if you start to doodle, keep writing."

That night I didn't have time for the writing exercise. With all the talk of abandonment, I thought I'd better spend some time with my husband. After dinner we put the kids to bed and went into our room for the evening.

He wasn't interested in talking about my therapy, and I wasn't interested in work, so we talked about the kids for a minute, then he leaned over to kiss me. I laid back on the down-comforter and tried to relax. The lust that filled his body with power, a desire that once stimulated me, was now repulsive. It had been weeks since we had been together and I felt guilty for denying his past few attempts, so I clenched my teeth and closed my eyes. His lips pressed up against my neck felt lecherous. The harsh dominance of his body over mine enraged me. I held my breath and tried to make him disappear, then exploded with aggression and pushed him away.

"Don't do this to me!" I lurched forward to hit him.

He grabbed my arm and held it down. "What's wrong with you?"

I looked up at him. And in the dim light, I realized it wasn't Phil holding me down. It was my dad.

Chapter 4

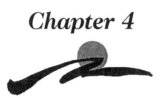

A nne greeted me in her office with a long embrace. My hands were still shaking from the experience of the night before. "Are you okay?"

I told her what had happened with Philip and how, after seeing him as my father, I'd jumped out of bed and locked myself in the bathroom.

"What were you doing in the bathroom?"

"I was just in there crouched down in the corner holding my head. The thought that my dad had hurt me just kept screaming through my mind." My voice started to crack. "I'm scared, Anne, I'm really scared." My arms and legs were trembling hard, as if the fear was shaking up from the deep fibers of my tissues. Anne sat down next to me on the couch, her hand lightly touching my shoulder.

"Whatever you're remembering is in the past. It's already happened and you're safe now."

"I don't understand this. I can't believe my dad would ever hurt me."

She watched me like a cautious mother. "We haven't talked that much about your father. I'm going to need to ask you a few questions."

I nodded as I tried to warm my hands, rubbing them up and down on the thighs of my jeans. Anne stood up and picked up her yellow note pad and sat across from me in her chair.

"Can you tell me what kind of relationship he had with your siblings?"

"Good. He wasn't an affectionate man, and at times he was aloof and gruff with all of us, but he was supportive and generous, and we all had a lot of respect for him."

"Do you know anything about his childhood?"

I told her I knew very little. He was raised in an upper-middle class family in Ohio and had two older brothers and a younger sister. Other than that, the only thing he ever told us about his childhood was how much he hated going to church. He said his mother used to dress him up everyday in a heavy, wool "monkey suit" and parade him past his friends to attend Mass in the Catholic church.

"Do you know his parents?"

"Yes, they came out once a year to visit. My grandfather was a gruff, short, little man. Kind of nervous, didn't really say much unless he was telling somebody what to do. And my grandmother wasn't very warm, but she was nice, and very refined."

"Do you know if your father was a pornography user or whether he exercised any deviant sexual behavior?"

"I saw an occasional X-rated movie around the house, and I know he liked to go to burlesque shows in Las Vegas, but for the most part he was a very unpretentious, well-liked, well-respected businessman."

Another surge of fear ran through my body and I began to tremor from head to toe.

"You're okay, Dawn, just take a few deep breaths."

"I think I'm going to be sick."

Anne pulled the trashcan out in front of me and then leaned forward in her chair, keeping a soft eye contact with me until I started to calm down.

"Can you close your eyes?"

"Yes."

I closed my eyes but didn't lean back in my chair. My body was still trembling.

"Unclench your hands and remember to breathe. When you're ready, try to imagine you are at the top of a staircase and at the bottom is a door. I want you to walk slowly down the stairs, open the door and tell me what you see."

"I'm still scared."

"It's okay. You can open your eyes at any time and see that you are safe and in my office."

I took a deep breath and imagined myself standing at the top of a spiral wood staircase. I slowly walked down each step releasing the tension in my body as I descended. At the bottom of the stairwell, I opened the large white door. On the other side, a 1960's version of my father appeared, his short thinning black hair greased and neatly combed back, his brown knit shirt falling around the waist of his nylon brown pants. He took me by my small hand, and suddenly I noticed I was a four year old remembering one of the days we walked out of my childhood home and went into his car to play. That day, I was wearing his favorite pink and white dress, excited, looking forward to the special time I spent with my Daddy. We walked out to the driveway and climbed into the front seat of his red Mustang. We both started to giggle as he unzipped his pants and took both my small hands and placed them around his erect penis. I told Anne what I was experiencing.

"Anne, this is fun. I'm laughing. Dad's laughing. It's a game we play."

"How old are you?"

"I'm about four. But he's not hurting me. He loves me. I'm very special to him."

"Tell me what else you're feeling."

"Happy, playful. I love my dad, and he loves me more than anybody else in the world. It's just me and him, and we make each other happy." I opened my eyes and walked around her office, relieved, elated. "Anne, this is what I didn't want to know. But he never hurt me. I know it was sick, but it was like I was playing with a little boy. He was just playing a game — a game to show me how much he loved me."

Anne shook her head. Her brow pushed into the ridge of her nose. "He may not have physically harmed you, but you were being damaged. Dawn, you were four years old and he was sexualizing your love. There are a thousand messages that go with that kind of attention and none of them are healthy for a child."

I was so happy that I had finally gotten to the bottom of all the despair that I wasn't even listening to her. I had been sexually abused. There was finally an explanation — an event in my life that made sense out the long, heavy months of inexplicable pain and suffering.

"Dawn, I want you to go home and write about this memory. Write with as much detail as you can remember and bring it with you the next time we meet."

I went home, grabbed a pencil and notepad, and sat on the floor in the nest. In large block letters, I began to write about the special relationship I had had with my Dad. The love I felt for him was intoxicating. Anne was right. I had no business being in a love affair at four years old, but, nevertheless, it felt good. It was innocent. He might have crossed some boundaries, but he didn't know he was hurting me. I'm sure he would have never done such a thing if he thought it would ever hurt me.

I wrote page after page about the fun we had together. Then I noticed a fear creeping up my legs and into my body. My hands and feet grew very cold. My limbs began to shake. The tone in my writing changed and the pen seemed to take on a mind of its own.

He hurt me, he hurt me, he hurt me. It wasn't fun. He tried to kill me!

Scenes of my father's red Mustang flashed into my mind. The red vinyl bench seat in the back, a blood stained white cloth, and my father's black leather belt on the floor in the car started to reel past me in greater detail. The lips of my vagina suddenly began throbbing with pain and a burning sensation came from the walls of my cervix. I dropped my pencil and called Anne. She picked up the phone as soon as I spoke into her recorder. I told her about the writing exercise and the scenes flashing in my mind. She asked me to come back in; it was Friday afternoon and she didn't have any more sessions scheduled for the day.

An hour later I walked through her door, holding my head as I paced the small office.

"This is crazy."

She took a deep breath. "What do you need right now?"

"I need to be safe."

"Nobody can hurt you here. You needed to be safe as a child and you weren't. But you're an adult now and now you are safe."

I pulled the trashcan in front of me and sat down in my chair, chanting to myself, *You're not going to throw up, You're not going to throw up.* Passing through a wave of nausea, I began to remember.

"It was the summertime, just before my fifth birthday. I was lying on the floor in the family room, watching Saturday morning cartoons with my brothers. Dad came in and handed me a dress to wear. It was a white dress with little purple flowers and, I didn't want to wear it. I didn't like dresses anymore; I knew what they meant and I didn't want to play.

Dad told me to put on the dress and to get into the car, that we were going to the store. His voice was low and angry. I didn't know what I'd done wrong, but I knew I was in trouble. After I put on the dress I found Mom in the laundry room folding clothes; my little sister was crawling all over her. I asked her if I had to go with Dad. With her back to me, she turned her head and snapped, "Do what your father tells you to!"

I looked away from Anne and stared at the wall. "We drove up the hill by the big white cross and then turned down a dusty dirt road that led into a canyon. He stopped the car, yanked me by the arm, and threw me down in the back seat."

"Do you know what happened after that?" she said.

I closed my eyes and held my head. *You're not going to throw-up. You're not going to throw-up.* "I can hear his voice. He's calling me a bitch. He's talking to me like I'm an adult. Like I'm a whore. He's a different person. This is so confusing."

"Try to stay with it." Her voice was clear, calming.

"I see him on top of me but I'm not in my body. My viewpoint is from the roof of the car, like I'm a speck on the ceiling looking down on us."

"Do you know what happened next?"

I opened my eyes. "He raped me."

There was a long silence, then I looked up at Anne. "I had to clean the car afterwards. There was blood on the seats from my vagina. It was my fault. I made the mess."

Anne's eyes looked torn between anger and tears.

I leaped up out of my daze, kicked over the trashcan, and picked up the door stop and threw it against the wall.

"He raped me! That bastard raped me! My God, how can anybody do that to a child? To their own child!"

I grabbed my keys and turned toward the door. "I'm going to kill him."

Anne jumped up and stood firm against the door.

"Don't fuck with me right now," I said.

"I can't let you leave here. Hand me your keys."

"I'm bigger than you, and I'm probably a hell of lot stronger."

"I know you are, but you're not leaving here."

Standing so close to her calmed me. I took a deep breath and walked around the room. *I'm going to kill you,* my father's low angry voice rang in my ears. I couldn't make it stop.

"Oh, no. I'm in the bathroom with him. I've said something to my mom. He's telling me to shut up or he's going to kill me. Oh, God, he hates me so much."

Anne sat down across from me, her eyes still glazed with a tear. "You didn't deserve to be treated that way. This should never have happened to you."

I sat down in the corner of the couch and pulled my knees up to my chest, nodding in silence as I continued to remember. After he cleaned the blood off me in the bathtub, he sent me to my room for the day. I wrapped up in an old yellow blanket I had pulled off my bed and crawled into the corner of my closet. I was lost in that closet. I thought I had fallen asleep and couldn't wake up, stuck in a dark place in my mind. Then I thought I was in some kind of accident, buried down deep in a dark long tunnel. It was the scariest feeling. I had no connection to life. All my senses were gone. I couldn't remember where I was, my name, or if I was even alive, until I noticed the beat of my heart. It was pounding hard and fast, first in my ears, and then in my chest. My heartbeat brought me back. It made me realize I was still alive.

I came out of my trance and rambled on to Anne. "I wanted him to forgive me. It happened right before my birthday, and I thought maybe he would give me a present to show me he still loved me. But he didn't. He wouldn't talk to me. I knew he didn't love me anymore, and it was my fault."

I got up again and paced the floor. "Oh, God, did you know this, Anne? Did you know I'd been sexually abused?"

"I wasn't sure. So much is going on with you right now. It's hard to tell where all of this is leading. How do you feel?"

"Shocked. Like the script of my life has suddenly been rewritten."

She sighed. "It hasn't been rewritten. You're just safe enough to finally read it."

Anne and I spent the next several hours talking. The puzzle was complete and the picture, as grotesque as it was, made sense.

"I was raped by my father." I said it over and over — in disbelief, in confusion, in a state of shock. I remembered words and pictures, but after my initial rage, felt no emotion. I had severed myself from the event and from the child inside me who had suffered the heinous crime.

"I'm not telling anybody about this," I said as I again paced the floor.

"You might change your mind about that."

But I swore in those hours I'd never tell a soul. The truth about my father would hurt too many people, and I didn't want be the cause of their pain.

"This is not your fault." Anne repeated the sentence a dozen times, but her words felt meaningless. If I talked, the damage would be coming from me, and I didn't believe anybody in my family would see the situation any differently.

The rain poured down on the window behind her, and the light of the day had dimmed to dusk. I had been in her office for hours and couldn't process anymore, so Anne and I just sat, exhausted, looking at each other. The events of the day, and the open-ended time frame had brought us to the intimacy felt by old friends sitting up by a late-night fire — the comfort so thick, the closeness so intense, neither one of us wanted to leave.

"I could stay here forever," I said, "but I should really go home."

"I'm not going to release you until I know Phil's at home."

I looked at the rain trickling down the window. Phil was en route from an appointment in LA; if he was stuck in Friday night traffic, it could be hours before he was home. I looked at the clock. I was in my fourth hour of therapy for the day and I could no longer justify the cost.

"Enough about me," I said lightly, trying to shift the tone. "Let's talk about you."

She smiled, "What do you want to know?"

"Do therapists have better sex than the rest of us who learned about it in the back seat of a car?" Bad pun.

"Not necessarily."

"What about you? Do you and your husband have the kind of sex that takes you to another dimension?"

She chucked but didn't answer.

"I want to hear that you do, so you can lie to me if you have to."

"Okay, then, yes."

I grinned and tried another subject.

"How many clients do you see a week?"

"Around twenty."

"Let's see...twenty times 85 dollars a session, times 52 weeks in the—"

"Why are you doing this?"

"Because if I annoy you enough maybe you'll let me go home."

"You're not going to annoy me, but I guess if you're alert enough to calculate my yearly income, you're alert enough to go home."

It was a bittersweet victory. The world outside looked dark and cold, and what I really wanted was to crawl up safe in her arms and stay with her in her office.

"I wish I could stay with you," I said as we embraced.

"I wish you could, too."

I walked from her office into a cold rainy night, a chill running through my body. I was going to have to tell Phil. For the safety of my nieces and nephews, I'd have to tell my mother, brothers and sister, too. Was there a chance that anyone would believe me? Or would I be the villain while my father played the victim?

In the morning I called my mom and asked if I could see her. She came up the next day and we went for a walk down the street. There was no easy way to start the conversation. I wanted her understanding, but I didn't want to take care of her feelings.

"Mom, are you sure you don't remember anything unusual about my childhood? Any events that stand out as strange?"

"Dawn, I've told you. You were an independent kid. You did things your own way, and whenever I tried to help you, you just pushed me away."

"That's because I was sexually abused."

She didn't ask by whom. She kept walking and didn't look at me.

"Mom, I was very violently sexually abused by Dad when I was five years old."

There was a long moment of silence.

"That's impossible," she said. "Your father would never hurt you."

"He might not have thought he was hurting me. Are you sure you don't remember anything that would have been a sign of sexual abuse?"

"No, Dawn," she said as she shook her head. "You always liked your dad."

"Do you remember how I use to leave with him alone, to go to the store or to his office?"

"Yes, but you two did that all the time."

"Do you remember what I was like when I came home. If I ever looked scared or hurt?"

Her eyes glazed over, as if she was going into a trance. After a long pause she started to speak in a tone that sounded as though she was thinking out loud.

"There was one day...and you would have been around five years old. You were in the bathroom with your dad. I heard you crying from down the hall. I went up to the door and asked if you were all right, and you screamed to me that Dad had hurt you. He yelled back that you just fell off the counter and he was handling it. So I walked away." Her finger pointed like she was talking to the air. "But I remember what you had on that day. It was a white dress with little purple flowers."

Oh, God, she remembered it, too. The father I created in my mind, the one who would never hurt me, was gone. Dead. "Had we just come from the store?"

"Yes, I think it was a Saturday morning…you two had just gone somewhere."

"Mom, I remember that dress, that day, and that was the day I remembered being sexually abused by Dad in the car. Right before he took me into the bathroom."

She snapped out of her daze. "Dawn, that's crazy. I've been married to your father for thirty-eight years. He could never do anything like that."

"I know it's crazy, but it's true. It's the memory I didn't want to know about."

"I can't believe this," she said.

"I don't want to believe it either, but don't you think it's strange that twenty-eight years later you can remember what I had on that day? Mom, I can't tell you what my kids had on yesterday. You knew something was wrong, Mom. You knew."

"Dawn, your father could never have done that. And even if he did, sexual abuse wasn't public knowledge like it is today. We would never have known what to look for."

"Well, it happened, and I think you should come in and see my therapist with me."

"No, no, that's not necessary. I'll go home and talk to your father about this."

My mother went home and I poured myself into bed.

Anne and I spent the next several weeks trying to connect me to my emotions. I was besieged with images and flashbacks but disconnected from my feelings. At night, I thought I was in my childhood bed. When my children cried, I thought it was me. My consciousness swung from the dim past to the present, and more often, I felt transported into the realm of the spirit woman. In those times, I still felt the pull, the feeling that my destiny was unfolding toward something worth suffering for.

As the flashbacks continued, the more depressed I became and I was still unable to cry. Anne thought I could get some relief if I could bring my consciousness from the roof of the car back into my body. We tried on several occasions, but my mind flew off into darkness, into a strange state of stillness, instead of coming back into my body.

After a month of failed attempts, we decided to try some body work, an adjunct therapy that had shown promising results for releasing trapped emotions. Anne had experienced this kind of therapy herself and referred me to the woman she used, a local body worker named Dee.

Dee worked out of her apartment by the beach. As I knocked on her door, she walked up behind me, a beautiful blonde, tan-skinned woman with a long hour-glass body that moved with such fluency she reminded me of a mermaid. We introduced ourselves to each other as she let me in, telling me she had recently left a job with a chiropractor to work on massage and study Eastern-style healing.

She washed up in a small kitchen sink then walked me back to the massage room, a converted bedroom that carried the aroma of burning incense. She handed me some towels and asked me to undress. I took off my clothes, wondering how old she was. Her skin looked too flawless for her to be much over thirty. Her eyes were as clear as a child's. I sat on the table and asked if she had children.

"Just one," she said. "She's about to graduate from college."

Wow, she has to more than forty.

"You said Anne Myers referred you?"

"Yes, I've been her client for a while."

"Anne would be good for you. The two of you have the same energy."

"The same energy?"

"You came from the same planet." I thought we all came from the same planet.

She covered me with a warm white sheet and pointed to an illustration of the human body that displayed seven energy centers called *chakras*.

"In Western medicine," she explained, "we gauge our health by blood pressure and heart rate. In many of the Eastern traditions, medicine is treated more holistically. The body is understood as a mass of energy, the flow measured by the seven chakras that lie on the surface of your body's aura, energy that shapes itself around the density of your physical body."

"Can you see a chakra?"

"Some people can."

"Can you?"

"Yes, they look like spinning wheels. Lie down and I'll show you where they are."

I was nervous yet intrigued.

"The first chakra is called the root chakra, and it's located here at the base of the spine. Its energy flow is associated with security. It registers how well we are grounded and is part of our survival instinct."

"What does it look like?"

"The root chakra normally has four spokes and spins with shades of red and orange. But yours isn't spinning. It looks closed."

"Closed?"

"Your energy system is blocked." She didn't seem concerned. "The second chakra is right around the pelvic bone, and it's associated with your sexual energy. This one looks closed, too."

I laughed. "I could have told you that."

"The third," she said, " is at your sternum. It's referred to as the solar plexus and it is your power center or your will. This one looks pretty good. In the center of your chest is the heart chakra. It's associated with love, compassion and your emotional being."

"What does that one look like?"

"It's shut. You don't spend much time in this body, do you?"

"Apparently not."

"The next chakra is here at your throat. It's associated with honesty, communication and creativity. It opens when we find our voice or creative outlet. The sixth chakra is between the eyes, sometimes referred to as the third eye. Yours looks pretty open — you must be perceptive."

"Is that the perceptive chakra?"

"It's associated with intuition, understanding, and vision." She moved her hand up to the top of my head. "This last chakra is called the crown chakra, and it gives us clarity of thought. It's also known as the spiritual chakra, like the light of an angel's halo. This one looks receptive, too. The guides must be working on you."

"Something's working on me, but its all very confusing right now."

She smiled. "Everything is always happening for the higher good."

I appreciated her optimism but couldn't begin to see how a child being raped could be for anybody's higher good.

"Just relax and let me get some energy moving through those chakras."

An hour and a half later, I was in a state of euphoria that took me far beyond any relaxation massage I had ever received. It was temporary relief, but it was worth it. I decided that as often as I could afford it, I'd come back.

In my next massage session with Dee, I told her about the abuse. To my surprise, she was as detached from the atrocity as I was. She didn't appear to be concerned with the realities of the physical world. Instead, she offered her spiritual solution to my troubles.

"Dawn, what you need to do is go into a deep meditation and enter your higher self."

I told her that meditating out of my body wasn't a problem, but staying in it was. She ignored me and continued.

"You need to go into your higher self and forgive your father. Send him light and love and you will be healed."

Higher self? What about my lower self? What about the part of me that had to function here on earth? She rambled on about a meditation to help heal my father. I clenched my teeth and stopped listening. My father's healing was not my concern; coming back to life so I could raise my own children was the only meditation I cared to think about.

"You were right to be angry," Anne said in our next session when I told her about Dee's advice. "You can't possibly forgive somebody who has harmed you until you fully experience the emotions caused by the abuse. If you tried to forgive your father now, you would just be stuffing all those feelings down even deeper." She looked enraged with maternal passion and it took her a minute to calm herself down.

"Spirituality has its merits," she said, "but not if it's used to avoid your problems or deny your pain."

"Don't worry — those were my thoughts exactly."

Her eyes took on the preoccupied look she had when she was carefully contemplating her words.

"I hate it when you do that," I said. "Just say what's on your mind."

She took a deep breath. "Dawn, the spirit you describe in your room, the increasing grace or coincidences in your life, even the vibrations you feel in your body — they are all the result of a process called spiritual transformation. There is not a lot of published information on this process, but it seems to be happening to people with a greater frequency."

"What's a spiritual transformation?"

"You are starting to become more aware. You're connecting to a deeper, wiser part of your being and embodying or bringing in a higher, more refined energy. The process changes your cellular structure and it opens your mind to new dimensions of your psyche. That's why I gave you Dee's name. The chakra system is an important part of the process; the energy that you're starting to release needs to be managed."

"Then what's with the sudden recollection of the sexual abuse? Why, after all these months in therapy am I just now remembering it?"

"A genuine spiritual path is often painful. In order to cleanse your system, your mind begins to release all the old memories, emotions and thought patterns that have kept you stuck in lessor states of awareness. It's a difficult process, but I promise you, if you stick with it, it will be worth it."

"It doesn't feel like I have a choice."

"To tell you the truth, you probably don't."

"Is there anything I can do to make this smoother?" I asked.

"You're getting your own guidance. The Indian woman has so far told you it's important to stay in the present. It's necessary to love yourself. And she let you know when it was time to know the truth about your father. Those were all good internal messages. The key is to trust them."

"Anne, it's hard for me to trust anything, let alone my own thoughts and perceptions."

"Of course it is. Your trust was brutally violated as a child, and your present world reflects your childhood. It's going to take time to correct old perceptions."

My brain felt like it was being reformatted. "This is all so disorienting. I feel like I've landed in the land of Oz."

Anne smiled. "Actually, that's a pretty good analogy for transformation."

"Have you done this work before?" I asked.

She thought for a moment. "I'd have to say I'm still on the yellow brick road."

I dished out the bad news about the abuse to one person at a time. I thought Philip's first words were going to be "I'll kill him." But the night I came home from Anne's office and told him about the abuse memories I had recovered, he looked like the weight of the world had been lifted from his shoulders.

"I've always known there was something wrong," he said, "and I always thought it was me."

My brothers and sister had mixed reactions. My younger brother Mark thought I was crazy, but my sister and older brother were more congenial. They had no memory of being abused themselves, but the fact that I was came more as a shock than a surprise. The shock was how to deal with it. We all respected my father, and his darker side was not one any of us wanted to see.

"We support you, Dawn," James and Kristen said on the phone, "but that was your dad. We had a different father."

My encounters with my mom were sadly predictable. The first month, I had her "one hundred percent support," but, by the next month, I had false memories, a theory she latched onto when dad brought home an article about a therapist who had led a client to believe she was sexually abused by her father. Dad made several copies of the article and told mom, "This article saved my life."

I heard nothing from my father directly. He told mom he was too angry to talk with me and refused to get on the line when I called. After a month of no contact I decided to appeal to his business sense, since this was the level where we were both most comfortable:

Dear Dad

Enclosed are the receipts from my therapy bills. Could you please help me out with the cost?

Love,
Dawn

A month later, and after mom nagged him to reply, I received a short note. Attached was a copy of the "false memories" article.

Dear Dawn,

I can not help you with the bills. The enclosed article explains better than I ever could.
I have to say a few more things.

You have been dredging up the past with bitterness and anger for the past seven months. Neither you, Anne or God can change it, but you can make the future.

You have fifty years ahead of you. Fifty years of books, music, children, travel, a marvelous and supportive husband, friends, triumphs and disappointments.

Let the past ebb away where it belongs, in the past. Get on with your life and live it with zest and fullness not clouded with bitterness.

I will always remain at a distance, wishing you well.

I crouched to the floor after I read his letter. Despite the abuse, I still loved my father, and I was crushed that he could end our relationship without any attempt to resolve it. After a week of trying not to believe my own memories, I sat down and wrote him a letter. I explained the symptoms I had had since I was a child. I explained how Anne had supported my recall but had never even once suggested that I had been abused. I closed with an open invitation to come to therapy with me and told him I was willing to work with him on a resolution.

I mailed the letter, but received no response.

Anne and I continued to meet twice a week. She rarely booked clients after my session, so if I wanted to stay a little longer, I could. It was a temptation I regularly succumbed to. Her responses to my questions were becoming predictable, but the only time I felt good was when I was with her.

I still did body work with Dee, partly because I thought I needed it, and partly because she worked on Anne and the mere mention of Anne's name made her ramble as though she'd been cast as a hairdresser. I now knew where Anne lived, had heard a few tidbits about her husband, and had been given a rather lengthy interpretation of her astrological sign. I was ashamed of myself for resorting to Dee's gossip, but I relished the access to information I wouldn't normally have had as a client.

My relationship with Dee helped me feel more secure with Anne, but elsewhere there was little stability. California was sliding into an economic recession, and our clients were dropping as fast as our relatives. Philip's daily reports were now given with a forced smile, so I modemed into the accounting system at the office and pulled up the income statement. When I reached the bottom line my heart skipped a beat. The company was as sick as I was, and I didn't have the strength to do anything about it.

I turned off the computer and sat back in my chair.

"What's next, God?"

A week later, I wished I hadn't asked.

Chapter 5

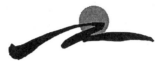

I tucked the kids into bed and went into my room. Phil was sitting up reading a book while I went in to wash my face. We hadn't spoken much that week; sometimes it was too painful to even make eye contact.

I crawled in next to him but stayed on my side.

"Are you tired?" he asked.

"Exhausted."

He put down his book and turned off the light. I rolled toward the window and let my mind wind down from the day. It was Thursday night. I usually saw Anne on Thursdays, but it was Memorial Day weekend and she and her husband had left early for a vacation in Oregon. I hoped she was enjoying herself. The work we were doing was grueling, and I was glad that at least one of us could get away from it for the weekend. Wishing her well, I nodded off quickly.

Let her go.

My eyes shot open. I sat up in my bed and shook my head. No, it wasn't a message, just my imagination. I lay down again and closed my eyes.

Let her go.

My heart began to race. I jumped out of bed and started pacing the floor.

"Let her go," I said out loud. "Why do I have to let her go?"

"What's going on?" Phil said.

I turned on the light next to his bed and sat down beside him.

"I just got a message. It was about Anne. She's going somewhere and I'm supposed to let her go."

Phil was adjusting to the absurdity. "Has she ever said anything about going anywhere?"

"No, she's never mentioned a thing. We had an agreement. She said she was going to see me through this. I can't believe she would leave. It doesn't make sense."

"Maybe it's not true." He turned off the light and asked me to get back in bed. But I was too unnerved to sleep, so I wandered into the nest and lay down on the bed there. Anne was restless. I had seen it in her eyes. Orange County just wasn't her style. She must have gone to Oregon to look for a new home.

I spent the next hour calming myself down. It would take time for her to move. She'd have to sell her house and close her business. That would take at least a year. By then I'd be better. A year from now, I wouldn't need her the way I did today.

Tuesday morning I walked into my session. Our eyes met as soon as I entered the door. Anne was sitting in her chair, silent, wearing the green leggings and the long, silk, button-down, leopard print shirt she had worn so many times before. I set my keys down and stood in front of the couch, a feeling of sadness hung thick in the air.

"So, are you moving to Oregon?"

She got up and closed the door. "Can you sit down? I have something to tell you."

The blood rushed to my stomach, my knees collapsed and I sank onto the couch.

"I'm not moving to Oregon, but I am leaving. Some personal issues have come up in my life, and I can't avoid them anymore. I'll be taking an indefinite sabbatical in ninety days."

"What?" Ninety days.

"Dawn, it's so hard to explain this, but my feet feel like they are being pulled right out from underneath me. I've been fighting it for a while now, and I can't avoid it anymore." She took a deep breath. "In September, Dave and I are going camping in Mexico for several months. Then we plan to travel through the States for a year or two."

"You're kidding me?" Mexico.

"No, I'm not. We decided this weekend, and you're the first person I've told."

I stared at her in disbelief, my head spinning so fast all I could do was nod. I picked up my keys and stood up to leave.

"Please don't go," she said.

I glared at her and walked out the door. The floor down the hall felt as though it was tilting to the left. My ears were ringing so loud I thought my head would explode. Ninety days. Indefinite leave. Mexico! There would be no phones, no mail boxes. In ninety days, she'd be as good as dead to me.

I leaned up against a wall and pressed my hands against my throbbing temples. Where was I going? Anne was the only one who knew how painful this was. My mind went blank for a moment, then I turned around and stormed back into her office. The door was open—she hadn't moved from her chair.

"How can you do this to me!" I slammed the door behind me. "You promised you would be here for me! You promised you would help me through this! It was our deal, your commitment to my healing. How the hell can you walk out on that?"

She kept eye contact with me but didn't speak.

"You asked me to trust you, and I did! You told me it was safe to depend on you, and I do! You told me you would be here for me and now you're not! Are you really so selfish that you're willing to re-inflict me with the same wound I grew up with!" I wanted my words to cut her, to stab her deeply so she would bleed as badly as I was bleeding.

She looked down at the floor and broke into tears. "I'm sorry."

My anger disappeared as I watched her cry. She looked so hurt, so vulnerable—all I wanted to do was hold her.

Let her go.

Oh, God, that's right. She did have to leave, and I had to let her. I dropped down in front of her chair and put my arms around her shoulders.

"I'm so sorry. I don't understand this, Anne, but I know you're doing the right thing."

She put her hand up against my chest and shook her head in tears. "No, please, please don't comfort me." Her arm went limp and I wrapped my arms around her back and pulled her in closer, my large green-knit sweater keeping us both warm. She released a deep breath that deflated her body, put her arms around my waist and started to sob.

"I received a message the other night that you were leaving and that I needed to let you go. It didn't make sense to me at first, but now I realize there are other people that need to come into my life and there are other places that you need to go." I couldn't believe what I was saying, or the peace of mind that came with it. We opened to a loose embrace, holding each others hands as we kept an eye contact that felt soft and loving — a connection I didn't know I could maintain with anyone other than my children.

"Dawn, this was one of the hardest decisions I've ever had to make. I love you very much, and I don't want to hurt you."

We fell into another embrace. "I love you, too."

My voice came from the center of my body. The sound of my own words stunned me, the tone much deeper than I had ever heard. I let go of my thoughts and absorbed the moment. How relieved my chest felt against the warmth of her body, as if I had finally connected to what I had lost — made whole again by a spirit that had enveloped us like a cocoon. She squeezed me tighter, as if a surge of love was going through her system, and suddenly my focus was drawn to my center, where I felt something I hadn't felt before. From within me, yet beyond me, there arose a small bubble of energy, as if the spirit that had surround us had entered my body — resurrecting my soul — igniting it like a small flame.

"I've never felt this before," I said.

"I haven't felt it for a long time," she told me.

I drove home without any memory of doing so, confused about my session, knowing only that Anne's sabbatical wasn't what I was confused about. When I pulled into the driveway, Phil was packing the car for Mexico. The trip had been planned for several weeks, but under the circumstances of the morning, I had completely forgotten. The baby sitter arrived a few minutes later, and I threw together a bag and jumped in the car.

We drove the next four hours in silence. Phil put on a pair of headphones. I stared out the window and over the Mexican waters.

She really did love me...but why? I hadn't done anything to earn her love. I didn't excel at a job that would command her respect. I hadn't even performed an act of sex to earn her affection. And she still loved me?

The emerging revelation was making me dizzy. The thought that someone could love me not for what I did but for who I was had never before occurred to me.

We spent two days in a cabin on the beach that we had been going to since we were in high school. Phil fished most of the time. I stared at the ocean during the day, the stars at night.

"You're starting to scare me," Phil said one night by the fire. "You're acting like you're brain dead."

I told him about Anne leaving. He shook his head and clutched his beer. He had interviewed Anne in the beginning of our therapy and had trusted her to care for me.

"I want to talk to her," he said.

"No. Don't get involved. I think she and I will be able to work this out."

He left the fire and walked down to the water. I crawled into my sleeping bag and stared at the wall. She can't leave yet. Our relationship isn't over.

Therapy with Anne wasn't the same after that. I was waiting for her to scrap our therapeutic relationship and move on to a friendship so we could stay in contact, but she didn't seem to have the same idea. We talked about her leaving and she'd slip into intimacy, then abruptly pull back into her role. "How does that make you feel?" was now thrown in rather than asked. "What does that look like?" sounded contrived.

I was as confused as Anne, but for different reasons. My childhood had been exposed. My family of origin had been dissolved. My marriage had been reduced to separate rooms, and I was in love with a woman who had no place in my life. I ran through the equation a thousand times. What did I want? What was I was looking for? Anne wasn't offering a relationship outside of therapy, and even if she had been, I wasn't sure what kind of relationship I wanted. I loved her deeply, but it wasn't the kind of love I wanted to share a toothbrush with. I didn't want to leave my husband or change my lifestyle. All I really needed was to stay in contact — to stay connected to the deepest love I had known.

After several sessions of waiting for Anne to make amends for our broken contract, I decided to take the initiative to try and resolve the situation. I walked into her office confident of the outcome. I knew she loved me, and I thought that meant that she would find a way for us to stay in contact.

"Anne," I said as I sat down on the couch, "I support your decision to leave, but my whole being is telling me our relationship isn't over. I know that sounds like I'm dependent, and I am, but I truly think this strong feeling is coming from a deeper part of my mind."

She looked at me softly. "It feels premature to me, too, but I still have to go."

"I know you do, but can't we convert our relationship to something else? Some kind of arrangement so we can stay in contact?"

"You can't convert a therapeutic relationship to something else."

"How come?"

"It's against the law. If I'm not your therapist, I can't have any contact with you for at least two years."

"That's ridiculous."

"I know you have a hard time with this, but there is a natural imbalance of power here. The law is set up to protect you, and I support it. I've seen too many people abused when therapeutic relationships are socialized."

"I don't want to socialize our relationship. I just want to stay in contact with you."

She shook her head and pressed herself back in her chair. "I can't, Dawn. You're the kind of person that goes soul-to-soul with people and...I...I just can't give you that kind of relationship."

"You already have."

She looked away and folded her arms, then looked at me again. The light in her eyes had faded away. "I don't know how I can make you understand this, but the therapeutic boundaries really are for your protection. It's the most unselfish thing I can possibly do for you."

"Unselfish. Anne, the boundaries are giving you a clear-cut way out of this relationship, and I'm stuck carrying the baggage."

"I'm not looking for a way out. In fact, if I had my way, I'd be taking you with me. But that's not in your best interest, and what's in your best interest is my first priority."

I felt like I was being strapped into a straight jacket. "Boundaries or not, this relationship of ours is happening on several different levels and it needs to run its course. If I could stop the energy behind it, I would, but I can't. It's bigger than me."

"I hear what you're saying and I trust your feelings, but I also know what I have to do."

I stared into the corner. Was she pushing me away because she cared too much? Or because she didn't care as much as I thought?

"Dawn, this is a bad time to be bringing this up, but there is one other thing I have to tell you. I have plans for a two-week vacation at the end of the month."

I laughed at her. "Of course you do. Everybody needs a two-week vacation before they go on their indefinite sabbatical."

"I'm sorry, but I really, really need to spend some time with my family." She looked liked she was about to elaborate, then stone-walled me by reasserting her role.

I stood up. "I can't do this anymore," I said. "There's a cadence to my process and whether you're here or not, it goes on."

"I can give you a referral for the two weeks when I'll be gone."

"No, I don't want to drag this out all summer. Why don't you give me a referral for a new therapist?"

There was a long silence, then she stood up from her chair and handed me a business card from her desk. "There's a woman who works out of the office next door. She has a lot of experience counseling incest survivors. I've put some thought into this, and I think her personality would work well with yours."

I looked down at the card, it read, Karen Edwards M.F.C.C. Her office phone was in the lower left corner. Her home phone was on the right.

"She puts her home phone number on her business cards?"

"I think you will find Karen is very available for her clients."

I picked up my keys from the table and stood tall in front of her.

"Do you want to set up our next appointment?" she said.

"No. I'll call you."

Her eyes welled with tears as I reached for the door. "Dawn, I know it's hard for you to believe anything I say right now, but please know there's nothing in the world I would like more than to grieve this loss with you."

I turned back and looked at her. My heart wanted to collapse in her arms, but my pride was back in control. I turned and walked out the door.

"Enjoy your vacation."

I came home and took the kids to the park. They ran off to the jungle gym while I sat on the edge of the sandbox, my teeth still grinding from the session. *You go soul-to-soul with people, and I can't give you that kind of relationship.* I wanted to scream. I wanted to cry. I wanted to push Anne Myers out of my life and prove to her I was never going to need her again.

"Mom!" Oh, God, the kids. There's Samantha...Michael. Where's Erica?

"Sam, where's Erica!" I ran around the playground, frantic, searching for my two-year-old. Moments of terror passed until I rounded the corner and saw her playing under the slide. I caught my breath. This relationship with Anne was making me lose my mind.

I made an appointment with Karen Edwards. As I sat in the lobby waiting for her to come out and greet me, I stared at Anne's door. It was closed, and there was no light coming up from the floor. A door opened next to hers and Karen walked out, a bob-cut brunette with a round, sunburned faced and a tall, confident stride. She looked younger than Anne, a year or two older than me.

"Hi, come on in," she said through a bright, white smile that wrapped across her face.

I rose slowly from my chair, walking back to her office feeling as if I'd been sentenced to foster care. She turned on the phone recorder while I stood in the center of the room. A light blue and white striped couch stood against one wall, a blue chair sat across from it, and the same bay window as Anne's office let light into the room. The room was bold and cheery; and if she was, I was leaving.

"So you're getting the double whammy," she said.

"Yes, I guess I am."

"Well, I want you to know that I'm here for you. What you're going through is difficult, and you don't have to go through it alone." Bull shit. I went through everything alone.

She spent the rest of the session trying to establish some trust. She told me she would meet me where ever I felt comfortable, then volunteered her schedule, numbers where she could be reached, and the location of her home. It was clear that the therapeutic boundaries were not going to be an issue. She presented herself like a trusted friend and I could see it in the way she described her practice. Her clients where mostly bulimic teenagers, kids she was trying to keep alive, too vulnerable for a rigid structure. After our session she walked me out to my car.

"If you ever need anything," she said, "just track me down."

Her efforts were genuine and I needed to move on from Anne, so I committed myself to weekly sessions, went home and wrote Anne a note.

Dear Anne,

>*It's time for me to get on with my incest issues and I'm confident that Karen will be able to help me through them. I would appreciate it if you could give her my file and any other pertinent information about my case.*
>
>*I realize that there is much to thank you for, but my feelings for you are still very unsettled. For now, I will leave you with what I hope is my final check and a promise that a more appropriate thank you will follow in the future.*
>
>*I hope you and Dave have a good vacation. As always, you will be in my thoughts.*

Love,
Dawn

I put the note in the mail and called Dee for a massage.

The smell of burning sage began to relax me as I lay on the massage table while Dee poured some oil in her hands and rubbed it slowly across my shoulders. We engaged in some small talk. When my intentions weren't obvious, I slipped in the question.

"Do you know what's going on with Anne?"

For the next ten minutes I heard about Anne's struggling marriage. How she had outgrown the relationship with her husband years ago and how her two-week vacation was a feeble attempt to rekindle the romance.

"Anne's really having a hard time right now," Dee said. "She's thinking about getting a divorce."

Her words took the breath right out of me. I loved Anne, and it was painful to hear that she wasn't happy.

I spent the next month in therapy answering routine background questions, dealing with another memory of my father molesting me in his car, and trying to hide my frustrations from Karen. The loss of Anne was tying me in knots and I couldn't understand why it hurt so badly, and felt so intrinsically wrong.

"I'd like to get your parents involved, if that's possible," Karen said in our next session.

"So would I, but they're not interested."

"Do you mind if I call your father?"

"Go ahead, but he's not going to talk to you. He told my mom that he's thankful for the thirty years he had me as his daughter and now he's moving on with his life."

"How does that make you feel?"

"I don't know. I think he feels that staying out of my life is the best thing he could do for me."

Karen's eyes never left mine. "Dawn, do you see any similarity between your relationship with your father and your relationship with Anne?"

"No. They're totally different people."

"I know they're different, but do you see any similarity in their actions?"

"No, and I don't want to spend money in therapy talking about my therapist."

She stared at me for a moment, then wrote down some notes. "Are you experiencing any more memories?"

I told her I was experiencing flashbacks, segments of memory that were becoming disorienting. When I closed my eyes at night, I felt as if I was a child, back in my childhood bed. Just the night before, a wave of terror had come over me that was so powerful I couldn't move. When I opened my eyes, it took me a few moments to orient myself to the present.

Karen continued to stare. "Have you heard of post-traumatic stress disorder?"

"I know it's common in war veterans."

"It's also common in adults who have suffered from child abuse. The shock of the trauma is postponed until the survivor is in a safe enough place to process the information."

"Maybe I'm safe, and maybe I'm crazy."

"Post traumatic stress can make you feel like you're crazy, but you're not. Your mind is trying to heal from the past, and I believe the night terror you're experiencing is trying to tell you something, trying to help you heal. Have you written about it?"

"I do a written dialogue with myself as a child, where I write her questions using my right hand and then put the pen in my left hand and let her answer. She's been telling me there's more, but I don't believe her."

"Why don't you believe her?"

"Because I don't want to. I'm sick of this pain. I just want it to be over."

She nodded. "I don't know what you have been told before, but there is no cure for incest. What happens to us in our lives is a part of who we are, and sooner or later, you're going to have to embrace this abuse and learn how to live with it."

I sank into my chair. My life felt hopeless. "I hate this."

"I know it's difficult."

No you don't and I want out of here. "Do you do guided imagery?" I said.

"No, why do you ask?"

"It helps me get through my fears."

"To tell you the truth, I usually refer my clients to Anne for guided imagery work."

My heart came alive. It was a way into see Anne without losing face.

"Oh really? I think I'll give her a call."

Karen looked perturbed. "I'm not going to attempt to tell you what to do, but if you have an appointment with Anne, I'll want to see you right afterwards."

"Okay, I'll call you."

That afternoon, I left a message on Anne's machine and she called me back just before dinner.

"I was planning to call you," she said on the phone. "I guess you got to me first."

My heart was touched by the softness in her voice. I could tell by her elated lilt, she felt the same. We talked about her vacation at Yellowstone — the places they stopped and the sights they saw. Her trip sounded more eventful than romantic. Her voice was calm but not at ease.

"I just found out Karen doesn't do guided imagery and I'm having trouble with a new memory. Can we set up an appointment?"

"Sure, I have some time tomorrow. Is one o'clock all right with you?"

"That would be fine; I'll see you then."

Philip walked into the bedroom as I hung up the phone, plopped down on the bed in his white T-shirt and jeans. "Who was that?"

"Anne."

"I didn't think you saw her anymore."

I felt like I'd been caught in a love affair. "No, I still see her sometimes."

He picked up a sports illustrated and opened a page. I had to tell somebody about this, it might as well be my husband.

"Can I talk to you for a minute?" I said.

"Sure."

"It's about Anne."

"Yeah, what about her?"

"I think I've fallen in love with her."

He turned the page. "It would be pretty hard not to fall in love with somebody who gives you their undivided attention every week."

"It feels stronger than that."

"Good."

"That doesn't bother you?"

He looked up at me like he could really care less. "No. Maybe she can teach you what love is. God knows I've tried."

I picked up my pillow and retreated to the nest, wishing I could feel the love I once felt for him.

Our friendship turned to romance the night of my sixteenth birthday, when Phil brought a keg of beer to my house and told everyone he saw that there was a party. A hundred people showed up, including an African-American, tow-truck driver who walked in my front door, handed me a bottle of tequila, and kissed me on the mouth right in front of my startled mother.

When the party was over, I helped Phil load the keg in his truck. We were both sober — usual for me because I didn't like to feel out of control, unusual for him because he preferred it.

We walked away from the windows and stood in front of the garage. I was waiting for him to kiss me good night when he blurted out, "I love you."

My skin began to tingle, not from the love but from the panic.

"Phil, I really like you, and I want to see you. But I don't love you."

He grinned. "You will someday."

I smiled but didn't answer.

"The very first day I saw you," he said, "when you were playing four-square in the seventh grade, I knew someday I was going to marry you." I laughed to myself. There was no way in hell I was going to marry this guy.

"Phil, that's very sweet, but I don't fall in love, and I'm never going to get married."

His grin disappeared. "How can you say you're never going to get married?"

"I don't want to be a housewife like my mom. I want to be a journalist like Barbara Walters. I want to travel the world and write stories about interesting people."

"I would travel the world with you," he said.

"That would be fun, as long as you know, I don't fall in love."

Phil's humor, intelligence, and persistence for my affection continued to charm me. And I don't remember the day, but sometime that year between the teenage parties and the sunset swims at the beach, it happened. I fell in love when I wasn't looking.

I walked into Anne's office like a teenager with a crush, so happy to see her I had forgotten why I'd left our last session angry.

"Did you miss me?" I said as I plopped down in my chair.

She smiled. "Yes, I did."

"Did you solve all the problems that you can't tell me about?" I asked.

"I'm working on them. But I want you to know this sabbatical is very unlike me. I like to know where I'm going to be tomorrow, next week, next month. I don't like it when things change so fast."

"I know what you mean."

"Yes, I guess you do."

She took a sip of her tea.

"I heard you and your husband are having troubles," I said.

"Where did you hear that?"

"Dee."

She gave me a perturbed smile. "You know, I have regretted sending you to her for a long time."

"She said you're thinking about getting a divorce."

"I'm doing everything I can to avoid that right now."

"How does that happen?" I asked. "Do people just stop loving each other?"

"I suppose that can happen. But I still love my husband. That's why it's so difficult." I wanted to ask more questions, but before I could, she changed the subject. "Enough about me. How are you?"

"Scared."

"What's scaring you?"

"When I close my eyes I feel like I'm back in my childhood bed. I feel a terrible sense of terror and I can't move."

"Is that what you want to do the guided imagery session on?"

"It feels like the right place to start."

The right place to start would have been with our relationship, but we were both avoiding that quagmire. She picked up her note pad and turned down the music. "Okay. When you're ready, close your eyes."

I closed my eyes and focused on my breathing. I was nervous. The space in my mind was like black fog and I feared what would appear when it cleared.

"Dawn, when you're ready, I want you to visualize yourself at the top of a staircase leading down to a door. Take your time and walk slowly down the steps. When you reach the bottom, open the door and tell me what you see."

The wood staircase appeared and with each step I felt myself going into a deeper state of calm. When I felt the flooding sensation of the altered state, I stopped listening to her suggestions to move toward the door and noticed that I was in my childhood bedroom. It was night, the room was dark, and all I could see was the light coming in my door from the nightlight in the bathroom across the hall. Then I heard the heavy footsteps.

"I'm in my bed...someone's coming in."

"How old are you?"

"I'm five. It's nighttime. It's the night after the kidnapper tried to get me into his car."

"Can you describe what you're seeing or feeling?"

"I hear someone walking up to my door. I'm scared. I don't know if it's my dad coming to get me, or the kidnapper." My throat was clamping shut, I was so frightened I wanted to curl up and cry. "I saw a shadow of a man standing at my door, he walks in slowly and kneels by my bed. It's my dad, his whiskers are dark and he's not smiling. He's angry. He whispers to me that he heard about the kidnapper. He says I've been bad and he's going to punish me for talking to strangers."

A sharp, dry taste came into my mouth. I could smell my father's sweat. My stomach started to wrench.

"Can you tell me what's happening to you?"

"No. It's too disgusting to repeat."

"You don't have to repeat anything you don't want to."

I stopped the memory and went back into the black fog.

"I'm not in my room anymore. I'm flooding in space and not scared anymore."

"Good. I want you to stay where you are and ask yourself why you need to remember this? What is the significance of this memory?"

Her question prompted a stronger focus, and suddenly, I felt my consciousness being sucked up into a spinning vortex. My head and body swooned as the darkness cleared, and a rush of energy, knowledge that came in a cluster of red, blue and gold light, burst into my mind.

"We don't really know who people are." The words had a will of their own, as if the information had instantly traveled through space and was now coming out my mouth. "Anne, this is about you." I repeated the message that burst into my head. *"We don't really know who people are. When I see your soul, I'll see my own."* My mind went dark and my body fell into exhaustion. I took a few deep breaths and realized what I had said. My eyes shot open and I stared at Anne. "I swear I didn't make that up."

"I know you didn't."

I sat up and tried to orient myself to the room, rubbing the skin of my arms, trying to get a sense of my body. Then I looked back at Anne, knowing her eyes had never left mine, comforted by her accepting nod.

"When I see your soul, I'll see my own. Do you know what that means?" I said.

"No, but I trust it. I had a strong feeling we were going to get something important today."

I looked around. Her office suddenly felt like a cage and I wanted to get out of that room and away from her.

"This message has taken me by surprise," I said. "I need to go home and think about it."

"I need to think about a few things, too."

Anne came over and hugged me good bye. "This is going to be okay," she said. "Really it is."

I couldn't leave her office fast enough. All I could think about was how dependent on her I felt. My spiritual path appeared to rely on my relationship with her, and I didn't like the feel of that. It could take a lifetime to see my soul in hers and, as much as I loved her, I didn't want to need her one day longer than I had to.

I received a call that week from Anjie, the office manager at ICON. Phil had signed up two big accounts which stabilized the company, but nobody knew what was stabilizing Phil. Most of the time he seemed to be handling our situation well, a husband turned super-hero, taking care of his family while his wife was ill. But then there where the other times, the times he vented his anger through some insane antic. Since I'd left work, he had fired the purchasing manager and turned his office into a bar, bought a python as a company mascot, and had taken the service manager's new motorcycle and ridden it up the stairs into the accounting office.

"I think he's finally lost it," Anjie said on the phone.

I put down a sandwich and sat down at the kitchen table. "What did he do?"

"Louis, the warehouse guy, kept messing up on his paperwork, so today Phil went downstairs and chain-sawed his desk in half."

"He did what?"

Anjie started to laugh, but I knew she wasn't kidding. "He chain-sawed his desk in half. It was a joke. Everybody but Louis was in on it."

"Let me talk to him."

Anjie put me on hold. It was five minutes before Phil picked up the line.

"You probably just called to tell me how much you love me," he said.

"That's exactly right, until I heard you chain-sawed Louis' desk in half."

"It's a metal desk. I only chain-sawed through the keyboard."

"You know, Phil, I think the labor board might have something to say about that."

"About what?"

"Management by power tools doesn't sound like a very safe method."

"Yeah, but I bet Louis won't make that mistake again."

If I knew anything about Phil, it was that he never asked for my help. He just resorted to something outlandish, usually a drunken binge that ended with him throwing up in my car, just to get my attention.

"Phil, you're under a lot of pressure. I know you don't want to go into therapy, but maybe you should reconsider it."

"Sorry, I don't have time to indulge myself in therapy. I have a company and three kids to take care of."

"Then will you please do me a favor?"

"Anything for you, princess." He couldn't have been more sarcastic.

"Bring home the financial statements and let's look at selling the company."

Phil came home early that afternoon, with the chain-saw, a six pack of beer and a printout of the financial statements. He drank the beer while we went through the numbers. The new accounts were keeping ICON afloat, but the recession had our receivables out so far we weren't going to make payroll. I didn't have the energy to come up with a solution. Phil no longer had the patience.

"Can't you ask the masters of the universe to lighten up on us?" he said. "I can't take this anymore."

"Neither can I."

I prayed that night for something to take the edge off. I didn't think it would work, but, then again, stranger things were happening in our lives.

At eleven o'clock the next morning my realtor called. I owned a rental property in San Diego with my dad. He had gifted his half to me after my last child, Erica, was born and I'd put it on the market. It had been listed for a year and a half, and my realtor was calling to tell me I had just received an offer. I couldn't believe my ears. The offer was good, the escrow would be short, and the equity would be enough to take the edge off — and then some. I called Phil with the news.

"This shit is weird," he said. "But I'm starting to believe in it."

"I still want you to sell the company," I said.

"I'm going to start working on that today."

In my next session, I told Karen about the abuse memory but not about the message. I still wasn't sure what it meant to see my soul in Anne's, and I was afraid if I tried to explain it to Karen, she would see it as some subconscious attempt to cling to Anne. I had already ruled out that possibility, and I didn't need my intuition undermined by some all-purpose psychological theory.

I spent most of the hour with Karen rationalizing away my father's behavior, speculating about his childhood and the abuse he may have suffered. She listened patiently, then broke through my rhetoric.

"Dawn, when you remembered your father coming in your room, what did you see, and how did you feel?"

"It was dark. I didn't see much other than the whites of his eyes. And the feeling was mostly fear. As soon as he entered my room, before he even touched me, I could feel his energy overpower me. It was like this dark, ominous force had come to suck the life out of me."

"When he was abusing you, do you recall having any other feelings?"

I stared at the floor. "I felt sick. A feeling of sinking disappointment."

"Can you describe that to me?"

"My heart, my hope, sinks into the pit of my stomach and disappears. Then I can't remember."

"You dissociate."

"I lose all hope, and then I dissociate."

She sat up in her chair. "The disappointment you describe from your father's abuse, do you feel a similar disappointment when you think about Anne leaving?"

"No. Why?"

"Because your father, as your parent, had a responsibility to take care of you, to protect you, and to support you emotionally. Don't you think that Anne, as your therapist, committed to a similar agreement?"

"Anne isn't hurting me intentionally."

"No, she's not, but the situation is re-abusing you."

I didn't acknowledge her.

"Dawn, what if this was happening to Samantha? What if she had been raped by the one person she loved more than anybody in the world? Kept it a secret from herself and everybody else and then finally, thirty years later, she had the courage to love and trust somebody enough to help her. Then that person broke their commitment and decided to leave. What would you feel for Samantha?"

Samantha looked just like me when I was six — her blonde hair, tall lean body and freckled pug nose. The only difference was our eyes — hers were still innocent.

"It would be unbearable to think of that ever happening to Samantha, but I'm not Samantha."

"What's the difference?"

"She's just a little girl, innocent, precious."

"And you're not?"

"Karen, I was never like Samantha. I was a bad kid, mischievous, aggressive."

"You sound like you think you deserved what happened to you."

"I know it's not logical to think that way, but I still feel guilty. And no matter how I try to change my thoughts, it's still there. It's just who I am."

"Who you are is guilt?"

"Yes... I mean no... I don't know. " I was pulling my hair out from the roots. "I need some help."

"I'm here to help you."

"No, not your kind of help. You're going to think I'm crazy, but I have this spiritual guide. This Indian woman who's helping me."

"That's interesting. How do you contact this guide?"

"Usually through guided imagery. I need to call Anne. She can help me."

Karen put down her notes. "Are you going to see the Indian woman, or Anne?"

"I know what you think, but my relationship with Anne is very complicated. I don't really understand it myself."

"I don't like this, Dawn, but I'll make a deal with you. You can go back and see Anne if you start thinking about the similarities between your relationship with her and your relationship with your father."

"If I have time."

I didn't care what Karen thought, and I wasn't about to taint my love and respect for Anne with the abusive memories of my father.

I left Karen's office and slipped a note under Anne's door. She called that night and we made an appointment for the following week.

Karen's door was closed when I walked into Anne's office; I was starting to feel as though I slept in both bedrooms but neither one of them was my own. Anne was dressed more casual than usual. She had taken a couple things home from her office and the room was starting to look sparse.

I sat down and offered her one of the animal crackers I was eating.

She smiled. "No, thanks. I talked to Karen last night."

"Yes, what did she say?"

"She said you're running into some problems with guilt." I was sure that wasn't the whole story, but I decided to let it go for now.

"It's like tar," I said. "I can't get rid of it. I was hoping the Indian woman might help."

"We'll give it a try, but before we start, let's talk about you and me for a moment."

"Is this going to hurt?" I said.

"I hope not. I've been thinking about our relationship and how we can maintain it."

I sat up in my chair.

"Dawn, there is no doubt in my mind that you and I have been together for a very long time. However, I believe we find what we need in this world, and in this lifetime, you found me as your therapist. I have to respect that there is a reason for that. I can stay in touch with you after I leave, but for your safety, it has to be under therapeutic guidelines."

"What does that mean?"

"For the first couple of months, I'm going to be out of the country. When I come back I'll give you a call, and if you need to see me we'll work something out."

I didn't like it. The inside of my body felt like it was being squeezed by a giant hand, but I didn't feel I had a choice. "If that's the only way I can see you, then I'll agree. But only if you agree to own your boundaries as your restrictions and quit trying to place them on me for my protection."

"I'm not sure I understand?"

"The therapeutic guidelines are your rules. They govern your profession and you are restricted by them. I don't believe that they protect me. And I don't want you to try to make me feel that I'm governed by them. I live by my own rules and I need it to be okay for me to feel what I feel for you and to be who I am."

"How do I restrict you from that?"

"Because of your boundaries, you won't give me a friendship, but you have mine. And you always will. If you ever need me for anything, I will be there for you. And while it may be inappropriate for you to ever call upon that friendship, your therapeutic guidelines should not, and will not, keep me from extending it."

She nodded. "I agree, and I'm flattered."

"Good, then let's do another guided imagery."

"All right, get comfortable. When you're ready, start relaxing your muscles and letting go of your thoughts."

I closed my eyes and relaxed into the black fog I saw in my mind. When I felt my muscles release, and my body begin to float as if I was lying on a rubber raft that had been safely cast from shore, I asked for the Indian woman to appear. The fog cleared to a light background and in the center of my mind was the Indian woman, seated cross-legged as she always was, her orange shawl still wrapped around her large-framed shoulders.

"She's here," I said.

"Take a moment to greet her and then ask her if she can help you to relieve the guilt."

Before Anne finished, the image of the Indian women disappeared and two side-by-side pictures appeared in the center of my mind. The first image was the death scene of me as a guilt-ridden monk, my soul rising above the flames. The next was a scene from my childhood where I was playing and laughing as a three-year-old, rolling on a green lawn in a clean white dress. My focus went to the image of me as a child and a message entered my head:

There was no need for punishment. You were, and have always been, as innocent as a child.

The images faded but left an indelible impression: the only spiritual being judging my sins was me. I came out of the trance with a lingering state of peace.

"Did you understand the message you just repeated?"

"Yes," I said. "It was clear that I was always innocent. And, it seems like my self-perceptions have somehow created cause-and-effect experiences." Pieces of the puzzle were coming together. "That's why it's so important to love myself. That's why history repeats itself. It's a cycle of thoughts."

She wrote some notes. "What is important for you to understand is that the abuse was not your fault. You didn't deserve it. It was your father's sickness, not yours."

"I understand."

"Good. I want you to go home and write this down. The information you're receiving is very important."

"Okay, but I want to come back. There are a couple more things I want to find out before you leave."

"That's fine. Dave is having some trouble wrapping up his work, so we should be here for another month or so." We set up an appointment for the following week and I left her office feeling lighter, as if an anvil had been lifted out of my rib cage.

When I pulled into the driveway, Phil and the kids were out playing in the street. They ran up to the car, and when I got out and bent down to pick up Erica, Samantha put her arms around my neck.

"Mom, are you feeling good today?"

I looked into the bright light shining from within her soft blue eyes. I wasn't only feeling good, I was feeling innocent. For the first time in my life, I felt as innocent as Samantha.

The summer was winding down. I had a list of items I needed to buy for the school year, which added just enough to my chaos to keep me from feeling any of it. Karen continued trying to make me face the emotional affects of the incest but, like the rebellious teenagers she usually worked with, I fought her.

"Dawn, I called your father last week," she said at the beginning of our session.

"Really? What did he say?"

"You were right. He said he wasn't interested in talking with me and hung up."

"How did that make you feel?" I said.

She smiled. "Not very good. I can usually get parents to help, but I don't think we stand a chance with him."

"I told you."

"What about your mother?"

"She won't come either. She supported me at first, but then she said if she believed me she would have to leave my father and she wasn't prepared to do that."

"How does that make you feel?"

"I'm too numb to feel anything."

"Do they still see your children?"

"My mom comes up to visit them once a month, but I don't send the kids to their house anymore."

"Did your children have unsupervised time with your father?"

"Samantha would have been the only one."

"Are you concerned something may have happened to her?"

"I can't even think about that right now."

She nodded. "Did you think about the similarity between your father and Anne?"

"I forgot."

"You forgot?"

"Karen, there's nothing to write. There are no similarities."

"Do you have any other sessions scheduled with Anne?"

"Yes, I'm going to see her next week."

"Good, because it's time you have closure with her."

"I don't need to have closure."

"Yes, you do. Your therapeutic relationship is over. You need to close it."

"Anne and I have decided to stay in contact."

"You and Anne can do whatever you want, but she's not your therapist anymore. That part of your relationship needs to be ended."

I glared back. "Have I ever told you how much I dislike people telling me what to do?"

"Dawn, you were abused by an authority figure. It makes sense that you don't feel safe unless you're in charge, but if you want to get better you're going to have start showing a little vulnerability in here."

She put down her note pad. "It would help our therapeutic relationship if you would end your relationship with Anne."

"I'm working on it."

"Good."

The day I was scheduled to see Anne for my session I awoke to a premonition about her travels. I had a dense, almost chaotic vision of Anne in Mexico and with it came a chilling sense of danger. She was going in the wrong direction, and for some reason I was supposed to tell her.

The message troubled me for the rest of the morning. I didn't want Anne to think I was trying to interfere with her life or, worse, think I was delusional, or so dependent that I was trying to manipulate her plans. But the premonition went beyond my fears. And the chill of danger stayed with me until I promised myself I'd tell her. Then, like the clearing of a rain cloud, it disappeared.

I walked into her office to regurgitate the message. I didn't think it would change her plans, but I wanted to wash my hands of it.

"Anne," I said, "you're going to think I'm losing my mind, but I received a strong premonition this morning that Mexico is dangerous for you. It's the wrong direction."

She looked interested but not concerned.

"Considering my psychological state," I said, "I'd take any message coming through me with a grain of salt, but the feelings wouldn't go away until I agreed to tell you."

She smiled. "I trust your instincts, but I'm still going to Mexico."

"Good. I like Mexico. I think you should go. And to tell you the truth I wish whoever was giving me your messages would dial direct. I have enough problems of my own to deal with."

She laughed. "Which problems are you dealing with?"

"Well, I can get strong feelings about your travel plans, but I can't connect to my emotions about the abuse. I want my feelings back."

"I think you do feel."

"Depression, isolation, and a lot of frustration, but that's about all. The rest of my emotions seem to be locked behind this plate on my chest."

"The grieving you've been doing for the past year is about your unfelt emotions from your childhood. If you felt all the feelings associated with sexual abuse at once, it would kill you. That's why you blocked them out in the first place."

"But I'm not a child anymore. I want to feel the pain and cry the tears, and I want to do it with you, while you're still here."

She nodded. "Where did you say you feel the block?"

"It's in my chest. It's the size of *home plate.*"

"We could try to go into the block in your chest and release it through another guided imagery."

"Whatever it takes," I said.

"Okay, but before we go into the block, I want to set up a safe place for you to go. Close your eyes and tell me when you're ready."

My mind was well cued by the influx of her voice and I quickly floated into a peaceful state of meditation. "I'm ready."

"I want you to imagine a long white path. At the end of the path is a gate. You are going to walk down to the gate, and when you open it, envision yourself in a beautiful garden, a sanctuary where you can feel warm, loved, and completely safe. When you enter the garden, look around and tell me what you see."

The image came up as she spoke, a cement walkway that led down a small hill into a canyon of tall trees that was fence off by a white picket gate. I walked through the gate and the scenery changed, I was in a garden of freshly cut grass, enclosed by tall manicured bushes that separated it from a dark surrounding forest. A small stream ran through the bottom half of the sanctuary. There was a white bench that sat on a lawn underneath a coral tree and several budding yellow rose bushes were scattered around the yard. In my mind I took a seat on the bench and, as I described the garden to Anne, the image of three women appeared in front of me. On my right was the spirit of the Indian woman, who hovered in a seated position above the bench. On my left was the spirit of Anne, her face softly shining, her body formed of light. In the center and poised to speak with me was a petite, wise and stoic woman, in a long, white, angular robe with a tall, pointed collar that rose up to the short-gray hair that covered her ears. Her image was powerful, magisterial, and I felt humbled and honored to be in her presence. I described the woman to Anne.

"Go ahead and greet them," she said, "then ask the women if they have anything to tell you."

The wise woman stepped forward.

There were others.

My chest deflated as if it had been punctured. I couldn't talk. The implication was devastating.

"Dawn."

"Yes. The older woman said there were others."

"Do you know who the others were?" Anne asked.

I exerted my conscious control. "No, I don't want to know this."

"Okay, just relax and ask the women what you need to do."

The older woman again addressed me. *Write the book.*

I repeated the message to Anne.

"Write the book. Do you know what that means?" Anne asked.

"No, but I want to get out of this trance now." The thought that there were others was drenching my body with a despair that felt like another death.

"That's fine, but before you come out, ask the older woman if there is anything else you need to know right now."

When I see your soul, I'll see my own.

I repeated the message, then the older woman gave me a message to give to Anne.

"You need to get going," I said.

Anne started to laugh. "I need to get going?"

"That's what she said."

"Okay. Tell her I'm working on it, and, when you're ready, bring your awareness back to the room and open your eyes."

I could feel the look of disgust on my face. All I could focus on was the thought that there were others.

"I have no recall of there being anybody but my father."

"Maybe you shouldn't take it literally. Maybe it had to do with another lifetime."

I knew it was in this lifetime, but I had enough on my plate. Anne was leaving in just a few weeks and I was afraid to open any more wounds.

"Anne, you were in the garden. Not your body, exactly. Your spirit."

"Figures. Even your images are literal."

I couldn't joke with her. My stomach felt nauseated, my senses dazed.

"Did the message about the book mean anything to you?"

"No. I don't know what I'd write a book about."

"I imagine it would be about what you're experiencing."

"I'm not writing about sexual abuse. Nobody wants to hear about that. Not even me."

"Are you interested in writing at all?"

"I once felt a passion for it, but after my journalism class, I decided I don't have the talent." Ever since college I'd been phobic about writing. My secretary did my business correspondence. Philip wrote our personal letters.

"I've read your letters to your family," she said. "I think you can write, and it seems to me that if you're trying to connect with your feelings, it would make sense to return to your passion."

I appreciated her encouragement, but I wasn't in the mood. The days ahead were looking darker. I had been through so much, yet it felt as though the process had only just begun.

Chapter 6

Phil had a business conference in Washington, D.C., and I went along, hoping to find a subject for a book. Politics was the only thing that still remotely interested me, and I thought the timely trip to Washington was more than a coincidence.

My fear of flying had somehow subsided. The flight was relaxing. Other than a small air pocket at take off, I had no apprehension. We landed in Washington in the late afternoon and spent the evening sitting in a garden hot tub on the grounds of the hotel. The cherry trees around the spa were starting to lose their leaves and the air had a clean, fall chill. It was the first time in weeks I had felt close enough to Phil to tell him I had received a message to write a book. I didn't tell him about the rest of the message; the thought that there could have been "others" was still more than I could tolerate.

In the morning, Phil woke up early and went to his seminar. I took a shower, put on a pair of nylons and a navy blue suit. The outfit reminded me of the confidence I once felt running my computer business, and it gave me more strength than the shorts and sweatshirts I usually wore at home. I filled my briefcase with blank paper, caught a cab to the metro and took the next train to the beltway. It was a beautiful, late September morning, and my problems felt as far from me as I was from home.

"You're welcome to sit here," said a slender young woman on the train.

I sat down next to her and asked her about the military uniform she was wearing. She introduced herself as Sue and told me she was in the army and currently stationed at the White House, as a nurse on President Clinton's medical staff.

"What are you doing in Washington?" she asked.

"I'm writing a book."

"Oh, what on?"

"Social reform." That sounded good.

When the train stopped, we exited with the crowd. I lost sight of Sue before I had a chance to say good-bye, then saw her waiting for me at the turnstile. She was standing at near attention and greeting me with a warm smile.

"If you have time," she said, "I'll take you through the White House."

I wondered what the catch was, but that didn't stop me from accepting her offer.

After getting me a security clearance, she walked me through the Rose Garden, where I noticed the massive number of security agents roaming the yard even more than I noticed the precisely-manicured landscape. We walked past the media room and were turning a corner into a corridor when a man coming from the other direction bumped into me.

"Excuse me," he said.

I bounced off his chest and looked up at his face. "Excuse me... Vice President Gore," I said as he continued his pace.

I turned to Sue. "That was Al Gore."

"Yes, he's tall, isn't he?"

I laughed to myself. My life was becoming so unpredictable. A week ago, I'd been debilitated by depression. Today, I was running into senior executives at the White House.

We walked up to the Oval Office. That night the President was giving his State of the Union Address. The door to his office was closed and you couldn't hear through it. I tried.

We went outside and over to the executive offices. Sue gave me a quick tour of the library, then walked me out the gate and handed me a pass that permitted me to sit in the House of Congress during senate hearings. I felt mystified as I accepted them. It was as if this modest woman on the train was an angel pointing me in the direction of my next destination.

I spent the rest of my vacation watching loud, over-bearing senate hearings and mulling around the House of Representatives interviewing reporters, congressmen and security guards about the lifestyles of our elected officials. After three days, I had filled a yellow notepad full of information that distilled down to two very clear conclusions: first, I didn't want to be in politics; and second, politics was not what I was supposed to write a book about.

The day after returning from Washington, I received another premonition about Anne. It was early in the morning. I had just awakened and was laying in bed when my eyes clouded with a vision of Anne boarding a plane — headed not for Mexico but for Asia.

I jumped out of bed with a rush of adrenaline. Asia was a lot further away than Baja. But, then again, what difference did it make? Either way I couldn't contact her.

I left a message on her answering machine and that evening she called me back.

"How was your trip?" she asked.

"It was fun."

"Are you ready to run for office?"

"No. I think God sometimes takes us places just to show us where we don't want to be."

She laughed. "Then this is probably a good time to tell you my plans have changed. I'm not going…"

"Wait, let me tell you. You're not going to Mexico anymore, you're going someplace in Asia."

"I'm starting to think I should be paying you. How did you know?"

"I saw a vision of it this morning. It felt like the right direction."

"I'm amazed, but I can't say I'm surprised. Do you also know I'm leaving on Monday?"

I swallowed hard as my throat started to tighten. "No, I didn't."

"Dave can't get off work right now, so I'm going to meet a girlfriend who's traveling through Thailand. I'll be back the first of December, and then he and I are going to Mexico."

She wasn't going to Mexico, but I'd let her figure that out.

"So is this good-bye?" I said.

"No. I think we should have one last session before I go. I'll be gone for two months. We might not get a chance to see each other for a while."

I dreaded the thought of saying good-bye in a session, but like my trip to Washington, it felt like one of those things that I was meant to do. We made an appointment for Wednesday afternoon.

On the day of our last session I showed up with nothing to say. There were no choices, no words of consolation. I knew Anne had to leave, but I couldn't help but feel like a casualty in somebody else's war.

The office was locked when I arrived. I sat down on the floor and leaned up against the wall. Anne walked up a few minutes later in a pair of shorts and a maroon cotton shirt that contrasted with the gentle glow that seemed to shine up from under her skin.

"Sorry you had to wait," she said.

I cracked a smile and followed her in. We sat down and she started to talk—something about her travel plans. But I wasn't listening. I just watched her. Everything about her was illuminated that day—her excitement, her fears, and her love for me.

She took a deep breath and settled down in her seat. "How are you doing?"

I didn't answer.

She nodded. "Would it be alright if I just held you?"

"Anne, I always want you to hold me."

She sat down next to me and put her arms around me. I put my head on her shoulder and rested my hand on her bare arm.

"Knowing you were here made this bearable," I said.

"Yes, I know what you mean."

I closed my eyes. The moment felt so good, so warm, but all I could think of was how quickly it would be gone. Our relationship was limited by time, by boundaries. And no matter how much I loved her, that wasn't enough to keep her from leaving.

"Do you really have to go?" I said.

"I think we both know the answer to that. If I stay here any longer, I'm afraid I'll just be getting in your way."

"You're not going forget about me, are you?"

"No. I'm not ever going to forget about you. You are very much a part of me."

She got up and took a picture out of her purse. "Here, I want you to have this."

The photo was a close-up of her in a denim dress holding a small white rabbit.

"Sometimes," she said, "when we get away from relationships that are as intense as ours, we question whether they really happened at all. I just want you to know I was here, and this was real." She sat down again and put her arms around me. I couldn't find the words to describe how much she meant to me, so I closed my eyes and traveled past my thoughts, escaping in her arms to a place deep inside myself.

"I love you very much," I said.

"I love you, too."

She held me tighter and suddenly the inside of my body felt frozen. I opened my eyes and looked at my hand. It was resting against her arm, but it didn't look as if it was mine. I moved my fingers to feel her skin; my sensation of touch was gone.

"I wish I could wrap you up and take you with me," she said. "Hold you in my arms where I know you'd be safe. But as much as I love you, I can't protect you from your past."

My past. I was finding it difficult to talk. "Karen said there's no cure for incest. Do you believe that?"

"No, I don't. You'll be cured."

"Are you still sure about that?"

"Yes, I have great faith in you — and God."

I was scared, unable to feel my body — detached from my voice.

"Anne, I have to go. But before I do, I just want to tell you that someday I hope you see yourself the way I see you."

"How's that?"

"There is something very special about you, and it doesn't seem like you know it."

She smiled. "I have a feeling that's the point of my trip. I'm going into phase two."

"There are two phases to this journey?"

"For me there are. But, knowing you, you'll probably do it all at once."

She got up and handed me a note while I stood by the door, frozen out of the moment.

"I'm going to miss you very much," she said as we embraced.

I felt as if I was enclosed in a jar — my hands pressed against the glass, desperate to feel the warmth of her body, suffocating from the lack of oxygen.

I kept my eyes on the floor and walked out the door. When I reached my car, I opened her note.

I believe that the thoughts of those who love you can make a difference. That's why I want you to know I'm thinking of you now.

I know it is time when we will not be able to see or speak to each other. First, that will be <u>temporary</u>. But secondly, I want you to know that I carry you, very alive, in my heart. And you can always reach me by doing the same. Now is the time to call upon faith and use it. Because what we have had, and do have, is very real and no one can take that from you, ever! I believe in <u>you</u>. You're going to be fine, I know it!

Love,
Anne

I went home and went to bed.

In the morning I awoke feeling as if a relative had died; you forget at first, then it all comes flooding back. Phil had taken the kids to school and the house was silent. I called a friend and got her recording, hung up and called Dee for a massage. She had an opening for a massage that afternoon. I made the appointment and went back to bed.

Dee placed a warm towel on my back, but my nerves were so raw the cloth was more irritating than soothing. She turned on some new-age background music and started working on my neck.

"I talked to Anne the other day," she said. "I guess she's leaving on Monday."

"Yes. Her plans suddenly changed."

"I don't think they were sudden. She's been planing to go to Asia for a long time."

I lifted my head. "What?"

"She's been planning to go to Thailand since the beginning of summer. She might not have told you because you were a client. She has a thing about that."

Anne had lied to me? Dee rambled on, "I've done bodywork on the woman she'll be traveling with. I have a strong feeling those two are going to become very close."

Anne had lied to me. And I was about to be replaced by her travel companion.

A shock of electricity ran up my spine, through my head. Everything in my body started to tingle as the room began to spin and a black fog in my mind threatened to engulf me.

Love hurts, it can't be trusted, and it always leaves.

I raced home and called Anne's office.

"I'm sorry, the number you have reached is no longer in service."

I slammed down the phone and threw a book against the wall. "Damn it! How did I let this happen!"

I went into the nest and rifled through my desk, found Anne's number and called her at home. On the second ring she answered.

"Did you lie to me?"

"What?"

"Did you lie to me? Had you been planning to leave the entire time and you didn't tell me because I'm your client?"

"Dawn, you're going to have to back up. Where's this coming from?"

The soft tone in her voice brought me back to my senses. I knew better than this.

"Awe...oh...I'm sorry... I just saw Dee. She said you have known you were leaving for a long time and you didn't tell me because I was a client."

"I don't know what Dee thinks she knows, but I assure you I told you right after I made the decision."

I was stuck. I felt embarrassed about my actions, frustrated by feelings I couldn't quite name.

"I'm sorry," I said. "There's something very strange happening to me. I didn't mean to call you at home. I'm sorry." I hung up.

My knees began to buckle. I grabbed my phone book off the nightstand and lay down on the floor. It took forever to find Karen's number, then three tries to dial it correctly. After I talked to two children and a maid, Karen picked up the phone. I tried to tell her what had happened, but I wasn't making much sense.

"Where are you?" she asked.

"I'm at home. I need some help."

"I have some free time this afternoon. Why don't you meet me at my office?"

"I can't move. I can't even see straight."

"How do I get to your house?"

I gave her directions. Twenty minutes later she walked through the front door, asked the housekeeper where my room was and walked upstairs to find me lying on the floor. She sat down next to me.

"What's this all about?"

I tried again to explain what I'd heard from Dee and my phone call to Anne.

"What were you doing over at that woman's house?"

"Getting a massage."

"Dawn, you were down there because she knows Anne."

My shoulders sank lower than the carpet. "How could I have been so stupid? How could I have let somebody in my heart like this? I feel like such an idiot."

She sat down on the floor next to me. "This is not your fault."

"Yes, it is. I shouldn't have listened to Dee, I shouldn't have called Anne, and I shouldn't have ..." I lost track of my thoughts.

"Dawn you are being re-abused, and that is not your fault." I turned away and stared at the wall. "Where are the kids?"

"Samantha's at school. Erica and Michael are at a friend's."

"Good. I wasn't sure how you were going to handle Anne's leaving, but to play it safe, I'd like to put you in the hospital."

"Hospital? I'm not psychotic. I'm just having a bad day."

"No, this is more than a bad day. It's a breakdown."

I clenched my jaw and stared back at her. "No, it's not!"

Dawn, I've kept my mouth shut while you went back to see Anne, but that's over now. She's leaving the country in four days, and when she does you're going to have to realize that there is no rescue."

"What are you talking about?"

"There's no relationship on the face of this earth that will ever rescue you or compensate for the pain you suffered as a child."

"I didn't expect Anne to rescue me."

"I'm sure you didn't, but there's a five-year old rape victim that lives inside of you and she's been hanging on to Anne for dear life."

The truth hit hard. If I had sunk any further I would have been in the room below.

"That child is still stuck in the closet waiting for somebody to come and make the pain go away. And it's not going to happen. Our adult relationships cannot compensate for what we didn't get as children."

"But the need for her is so strong."

"Because it's an old need, a childhood need. You have to allow yourself to feel the pain of that need not being filled, and you do that by being true to yourself — and honest about your relationship with Anne."

"I was honest."

"Dawn, you've been using the facade of therapy to go back and see her all summer."

"Being a client was the only way I could see her."

"So, instead of suffering the pain of the loss, you became something you weren't in order to get something you needed."

"It's more complicated than that."

"When we change ourselves to fit somebody else's ideals or parameters, we are not being true to who we are in the world."

"Anne wasn't going to change her parameters for me."

"Then have the strength to walk away."

Tearing out the inside of my body would have been less painful. "I don't know if I can do that."

"You don't have a choice anymore."

Tears rolled down my face. The release felt like the first drops off an iceberg.

"Dawn, its time you acknowledge your losses and feel your pain."

"That could last forever."

"Not if you really feel it. And if you do, then eventually the pain will go and you will learn to see life in a different way."

I pulled my knees to my chest. "This hurts so bad."

"It's supposed to hurt. You've had more losses this year than most people could tolerate. It's going to take some time to work through them, and the hospital has a good program to help you do that."

"I'm not going into the hospital."

"I'm going to recommend the out-patient program. You can come home at night."

I tried to get up, but the dizziness sent me back down.

"What do you do there?"

"You'll spend the day in small therapy groups."

"I don't want to talk to other people."

"Everybody says that, but you'll be better off in a group than you will be sitting here in your room curled up on the floor."

"How long do I have to be there?"

"I going to recommend you stay for six weeks."

Karen asked to use the phone. "In order to be admitted to the program you need to be under the care of a psychiatrist. I'm setting you up an appointment to see Dr. Smith."

"Will I still see you?"

"Don't worry, I'm not letting you out of my sight."

That night I received a phone call from Anne. Her voice made me feel a hundred pounds heavier.

"Hi. I called Karen, and she said it would be all right if I gave you a call."

I hated that she thought she needed permission.

"I'm sorry about what happened to you today," she went on. "I want you to know I support your decision to go into the hospital."

"You must think I'm crazy."

"No." There was a pause. "Dawn, I don't judge you. I just love you."

I started to cry.

"I'm getting in your way," she said. "Karen is taking good care of you. I need to turn this over to her and trust that what's happening is for the best."

"Anne, this isn't your fault. Go and have a good time. I'll be all right." There was a long silence. "I need to get some sleep now," I said.

"Okay. Please take good care of yourself."

"I will."

I hung up, rolled up in a blanket, and cried myself to sleep.

In the morning I dragged myself out of bed to make my nine o'clock appointment with Dr. Smith. When I walked in the door, his secretary greeted me with a clipboard full of paper work. I sat down in the small lobby, scratched my name and address on the form and drew a line down the NO column on medical history. Then I handed it back to the secretary. "Excuse me," she said, "you didn't fill in your phone number." I panicked. They were going to slam me in the over-night program if I couldn't remember my phone number.

"My number is...is...is that important?"

She looked at me until I spit out the numbers.

"Doctor Smith will be right with you."

Doctor Smith was a well-dressed man with a short-trimmed beard who looked more like a young surgeon than a psychiatrist. We walked back to his office and went over my history. After the intake was over, he became less formal.

"Let me tell you a little bit about my background so we can get to know each other."

I stood up to leave. "I don't want to know about you. I don't want to care about you. I don't even want to talk to you." I swallowed hard. "All I need from you is your signature on this stupid piece of paper so I can be admitted to the hospital and recover from this nightmare."

"I see you don't have any problems asserting yourself."

"No, I don't."

He took a pen out of his pocket. "Dawn, I'll enroll you in the program, but I'll have to see you for at least thirty minutes a week."

I didn't like my options, but the hospital program was beginning to have that beckoning feel — the pull in my chest that told me it was someplace I had to go, to uncover something I'd need to heal. I agreed to his thirty-minute sessions and set up an appointment to meet him on Monday.

I came home and went to the nest, laid on the floor until the kids came home, then directed them to start packing. We had planned to go to Sea World for the weekend. The hotel was paid for, and I wanted them to go without me.

Phil came home and packed the car.

"Are you sure you want us to leave?" he said.

"Yeah, they don't need to be around me like this."

"I don't feel right leaving you."

"I'll be fine."

"Okay, but I'm going to call you twice a day."

"Please don't. I promise, I'll be fine."

They all kissed me goodbye and jumped in the car. I walked back in the house and locked the door behind me. The sun was coming through the living room window like a light shining down on an open casket. I lay down on the carpet and let the heat beat down on my face, then looked across the room to the picture of the Indian woman above the mantle. There was no sense of her presence. No images in my mind. The world had gone dark and I was alone.

I turned over on my stomach and watched a spider crawl up the baseboard. I could kill that bug with the flick of a finger. I could kill myself as easily.

I thought of the gun at the top of Phil's closet. My relief was a bullet away, and it had the added benefit of revenge. My death would be the cry my parents never heard. The only way I could communicate to Anne how much her leaving was hurting me.

I walked upstairs and pulled down the revolver, sat down at my desk and caressed the cold steel handle. I'd go into the canyon. The coyotes would eat my body, so there wouldn't be much to find. I picked up a pen. I'd write a note to Phil and then one for the kids. No, I should write each of them a note. Maybe I should just write one note. No, I'd tell Phil where I went. I'd just tell the kids that I loved them, but ...but what? What was I going to tell my children. *Sorry, I can't handle the pain. You take it.*

I tossed down the pen and lay back down on the floor. The pain was mine and there could be no revenge. My parents and Anne would blame my death on each other. My childrens' suffering would far surpass theirs.

I listened to Michael's iguana scratching the cage; it had more life in it than I did. If only I were a lizard, or a whale. Whales didn't leave other whales. At least not on purpose.

My digital clock flipped a number, and I thought of a young man I'd seen walking on the beach. I had watched him waste away, probably a victim of AIDS. The numbers on my clock meant nothing to me, but to him they were everything.

I should pick myself up off this floor and appreciate all the things that I did have. A nice home, my family and my health. Why couldn't I kill myself? Oh, yeah, the kids.

On Saturday, I moved to a new spot on the carpet. I should get a job. Get out of my head and stay busy with a career. Let's see what could I do? Sales, computers, accounting... forget it. How could I work? I didn't have the strength to take a shower. Maybe she'd call. No, she wasn't going to call.

By Sunday morning, I was disgusted with myself. I hadn't changed my clothes, brushed my teeth or as much as opened a window in the house. The kids would be home soon and I couldn't go on like this. I'd grieve Anne's loss until Monday morning. Then I would put this relationship behind me and get on with my life.

Chapter 7

Monday morning, Anne Myers boarded a plane to Thailand, and I went into a six-week outpatient program at the local psychiatric hospital. I woke up early and put on my jeans, a black turtleneck, and my ankle-high boots. The outfit gave me power — otherwise I felt like hell.

The hospital was a few miles from my house. I drove up early and walked around the spacious grounds, a series of one-story stucco buildings sprawled through an old eucalyptus grove that covered the area in leaves. The trees towered over the compound. Fields of long-stemmed wildflowers separated the buildings.

I walked down a path to the center court, a grassy bluff with a gazebo that overlooked Dana Point Harbor. I stood for a moment and watched a sailboat leave the jetty. The view was in black and white — a picture I couldn't taste, touch or feel.

Dr. Smith met me in the main building and led me into a small, sterile conference room with a wooden table and two metal chairs. I kept my hands in my jeans and pulled my chair out with my boots.

"How are you feeling this morning?" he said.

"I'm fine."

"I talked to Karen this weekend. She said you and Anne were very close."

"My being here has nothing to do with Anne."

"I know Anne. She's a good therapist."

"I'm not here to talk about my therapist. I'm here to recover from child abuse."

He looked at me while he rubbed his short black beard. "Dawn, if you cared for Anne and you trusted her to care for you, then I imagine having her leave the country in the middle of your therapy would be very difficult."

"It was, but it's not now. I've accepted that she had to leave and now I'm getting on with my life."

"Just like that?"

"Yes, just like that."

I got out of my chair and leaned against the wall.

"Do you see any similarities between the abandonment you felt from your parents and Anne leaving your therapeutic relationship?"

"Look, my dad was sick and he mistreated me. My mother was too naive to know any better. And Anne had a life to lead. I was just a client."

He nodded. "That's interesting. Who's protecting you?"

"What do you mean?"

"While you're protecting your father, your mother, and Anne, who's protecting you?"

"The only person who can... me."

"Then why don't you start by realizing that whether it was intentional or not, all of these people have hurt you, and if you ever want to get out of this depression, you're going to have to stop rationalizing away their actions and start to feel some of the pain it's causing you. I think the best place to start is your relationship with Anne."

"She's gone! I don't care about her anymore. Let's just get on with the child abuse issues." I kicked my chair, tears streaming down my cheeks.

"Why are you crying?"

"You frustrate me! Is this session over yet?"

"In a minute. Karen wanted me to review you for an antidepressant. I have decided not to put you on one."

"Why?"

"Medication is not a cure. It only treats symptoms and you don't strike me as somebody who is interested in managing symptoms."

"I just want to be well."

"It may be more difficult, but I think an antidepressant would just slow you down."

"Fine, I didn't want to take one anyway."

He stood up. "I'll give you a few minutes alone, then I want to introduce you to Stacy. She's the therapist in charge of the program."

When he left I fell apart, tears streaming down my face like large drops of rain. After a hard cry, I composed myself to be introduced to another therapist I didn't want to meet.

Stacy stood taller than I. She was an attractive, dark-haired Nordic-looking woman in her late thirties who had the strong, full body of an athlete. She extended her hand as we were introduced. With her firm grip and slight nod she let me know she was in charge – and if I didn't give her any trouble, she wouldn't make my stay at the hospital miserable.

After Doctor Smith left, we sat down and went over my history. Her questions were to the point, my answers brief. After the intake, she walked me down the hall and into a therapy group to meet the other patients.

The meeting room was small, with straw colored grass-cloth walls and no windows. Five chairs and a couch were grouped around an old, narrow-legged coffee table, set on a white-speckled linoleum floor that reminded me of my childhood bathroom. I sat down on the couch next to a woman wearing a long-sleeved white shirt and a pair of jeans, her jaw muscle was clenched so tight it extended beyond her ears. I said hello. She stared at a wall and jiggled her foot up and down on the floor.

The three women across from me were more congenial. We smiled at each other as Stacy began the group discussion.

"We have a new member today." Stacy introduced me and then asked the group to share what they wanted to about why they were there.

Liz, a petite, well-dressed woman with short, graying hair and a pale, brazen face, spoke up first. She told the group she was a senior vice president for IBM. "I had a nervous breakdown on a flight to New York," she said. "Other than that, I grew up in a slum in Texas, got married to put myself through college, and became suicidal after my last promotion."

"Why's that?" I asked.

She showed me the palm of her hand. "This is where my mother used to put out her cigarettes." I glanced at the deep disfiguring scars. "I've been working my whole life just to prove I was worth more than an ashtray."

The woman next to her was Mary, a short-round, middle-aged Hispanic woman who worked as a secretary in Santa Ana. Tears wrapped in heavy black mascara rolled down her checks as she spoke of being sexually abused as a child by her father and uncle. "My panic attacks turned into agoraphobia," she said as she clicked her bright red porcelain nails against the chair. "This is the first time I've been out of my house in six months."

Next to me on the couch was Patty with the tight jaw, a masculine looking woman in her late twenties with flaky, white skin, and fine, brown, hair cut short past her ears and then long and layered in back. She said hello in a low hoarse voice, but she didn't look at me, and she didn't say why she was there.

Stacy began the morning group by reading a meditation out of a small book. The book was passed around the room and each member commented on what the meditation meant to her. I wasn't sure if it was rigged or a coincidence, but the meditation of the day was entitled "The pain of loss."

When the book made its way to Patty, the pace of her foot accelerated.

"Pass," she said as she handed me the meditation.

"You can do that?" I said to Stacy.

"Maybe she doesn't have anything to share," Stacy said.

I looked at the book. "The pain of loss. I don't think I have anything to share either."

Stacy looked at me. "What about your therapist?" she said. "I understand she left today on sabbatical."

I could feel the eyes of the other members on me.

"Yes, she did."

"Do you want to talk about that?"

I stared at the table.

"There really isn't anything to talk about. I just came to trust, and, I guess, to love her very deeply. It was a special relationship."

Liz started to laugh. "Dawn, everybody falls in love with their therapist. It's the oldest one in the book."

"It is?"

"Yes. They're like objects we mold to fit our needs. We create them by imagining they're everything we ever needed in a person. It happens all the time."

I shook my head. "No, it wasn't like that. I know she cared for me just as much."

"You think your therapist loved you?" Liz said.

"Yes, I do."

"Dawn, what makes you think that?" Stacy said.

"She told me." I regretted the words as soon as they left my mouth.

"Your therapist told you she loved you!" Liz said.

"It sounds like some emotional boundaries were crossed," Stacy said. "Does your new therapist know about this?"

"These damned therapists are always abusing their power. You ought to report her for that," Mary said.

Report her? Why would I want to report her?

"That's all I have to say." I handed the book to Stacy and sank into the couch.

Everybody falls in love with their therapist. Great. I wasn't just an idiot, I was a common idiot.

The morning session was followed by lunch, an anger management class, another group process meeting, and then closing comments. At four o'clock, we went home. At nine o'clock each morning, we met in the same small room.

By the end of the week we were as cohesive as war vets. Liz and I were probably the closest, our contempt for authority figures the common bond. Patty was the only group member who hadn't participated. Each day she sat next to me, her leg crossed in my direction, her foot shaking like the little plastic toys you wind up to jump around the floor. By the end of the week, the vibration on the couch was driving me crazy. Out of sheer irritation, I found the nerve to grab her tennis shoe.

"Why are you here?" I said.

She looked at me for the first time. "I'm a cutter."

"What's a cutter?"

She pulled up her sleeve and showed me the deep, red grooves that lined her arm.

"Sometimes I can't feel my body. The only way I can tell if I'm still alive is to cut my arm until I feel pain." She pushed down her sleeves. "I'm also a lesbian and a bulimic, if that helps you any."

"You mean you actually make yourself throw up?"

"No, I can do it by will. Want to see?"

"No thanks." There was a brief pause before the more compelling question jumped out of my mouth. "So how come you're a lesbian?"

She smirked. "Because the idea of putting some guy's dick inside of me makes me want to vomit."

"Is that how you throw up at will?"

She smiled and befriended me with a nod. "Believe me, being a lesbian isn't a sexuality anybody wants to sign up for."

"Why not?"

"Are you kidding? You're ostracized from society, it's not easy to have children, and imagine how difficult it would be to be in love with a woman who has as many emotional needs as you do. You guys with husbands have it easy. All you have to do is hand them a beer and turn on a football game."

She got up and poured herself some coffee.

"Do you ever wish you were straight?" Liz said in her IBM executive tone.

"Hell, no! Men are simple, but they're still hairy, disgusting pigs."

Liz and I looked at each other and smiled. "I think my husband's a pig. Does that mean I'm a lesbian?" Liz said.

"Yeah, and I fell in love with my therapist, does that mean I'm a lesbian?"

Patty stirred her coffee, opened the door, and looked at us. "You guys aren't gay. You're just fucked up."

Liz and I looked at each other and laughed. It was the best diagnosis either one of us had received.

I came home that evening. Phil was sitting in front of the television drinking a beer and watching a football game. He grabbed my hand when I walked in the family room.

"It's fourth down, the 49ers are on the fifty-yard line. They're losing by six points. This play could be crucial!"

I put my arm around him. "Where are the kids?"

"They just went up stairs with Malagro. Can we talk at the commercial?"

I kissed him good night, appreciating how simple he really was.

On Monday, a teenager named Denise was added to our group. She was a tall, gangly red-head with cream-white skin and a tattoo of a vampire peering out from the side of her leg. Denise, wearing a pair of dark glasses sat against the wall sucking an unlit cigarette.

"Could you please join the group?" Stacy said to her.

Denise took a chair and kicked her feet up on the coffee table.

"I don't need to be here," she said.

"Then why are you?" Liz asked.

"Because I wanted to commit suicide, so my parents stuck me in this place."

"Do you still want to kill yourself?" Stacy asked.

"No, my doctor put me on some drugs and now I'm fine. There's nothing wrong with me. I just had a chemical imbalance."

I held back my laughter. It was good to see how far I had come.

"Your records show you have an IQ in the 140's," Stacy said, "yet you've been thrown out of several schools. How do you explain that?"

"School sucks. It's just a bunch of assholes telling you what to do."

Then again, maybe I hadn't come that far.

"You obviously don't like that."

She sucked on her cigarette.

"Have you tried challenging yourself in other ways?" Stacy asked.

"I write music."

"That sounds productive."

"Not if you write it on the side of a building."

We started to laugh. If the rest of us hadn't done something similar in high school, we'd at least had the inclination.

On Tuesday, we walked to another building for a group called Psychodrama. Stacy had warned us that the therapy was intense, a reenactment of a patient's abuse that often rippled through the group like the lancing of a collective wound. Because of the intensity of the session, the group mostly consisted of the day-patients and the adolescent unit. In-patients were considered too fragile to attend.

Our group was the first to enter the large, blue-carpeted room with 50 chairs encircling a stage. We took our seats. Patty was telling Liz and me about a fight she had been in with her girlfriend when the door opened and forty adolescents cascaded through the room. They strutted by us without a glance in our direction. We watched them as if they were creatures in a zoo. They had demon-like tattoos on baby soft skin, and ring holes on facial features that were still growing. The youngest of them could not have been more than nine. And beneath the hardening expressions on their faces, the precious glow of life still shone through.

Stacy introduced herself as the psychodrama director, gave a brief description of what the session would entail and then asked for a volunteer.

Several of the adolescents raised their hands. Stacy circled the room and chose a Latino girl, a teenager with large brown-eyes, smooth dark skin and a mane of hair that ran the length of her oversized flannel shirt. Stacy took her by the hand and walked with her around the circle.

"Could you tell us your name and how old you are?"

"My name's Maria. I'm fourteen years old."

"And why were you admitted to the program?"

"Da courts, they send me here, 'cause I helped to kill someone."

"Why did you want to kill somebody?

She smiled at a friend as she passed her.

"I'm a gangbanger. We have to kill people to get into the gang."

"Can you tell us what a gangbanger is?"

"Gangbangers are like me. We hate ourselves and we hate other people, so we kill them."

Liz looked at me. I just shook my head.

"I do drugs a lot too."

"What do you take?"

"Speed, crack, LSD."

"Are you clean now?"

"Yeah. I haven't taken drugs in a month."

They continued to walk the circle. "Can you tell us a little bit about your family?"

"When I'm not in jail, I live with my dad. He hates me because I'm in the gang." She stared at the ground, twisting her shirt. "He hits me a lot, calls me a slut."

"Do you have a mother?"

"She's dead. I have two sisters. They have jobs and go to church. They want me to live with them, but they live far away. I don't want to leave my friends."

Stacy asked Maria to pick some people out of the audience to play the influences in her life. Maria chose two fair-skinned boys and a girl to play the gang members, a strong stocky counselor from her unit to play her father, a handsome seventeen-year-old boy to play the seduction of drugs, and two Latino girls to play her sisters.

Stacy and three staff members placed each group in a different part of the circle and stood behind the participants directing their actions and dialogue. When everyone was situated, the drama began.

"You're a slut, Maria!" yelled the counselor who played her father. "A worthless slut, and you're not going to leave this house!"

The kids playing the gang members shuffle around her. "Come with us, Maria. We'll be your family — nobody else cares for you."

"Come with me," whispered the drugs in a low seductive voice. "I'm ecstasy, I'll take you away. I'll make you feel better than you have ever felt before."

Her sisters cried out from the corner of the room, "Please, Maria, come back, come to us, we love you, we can help you, give you a home."

"Be in the gang, be one of us, nobody else cares for you. We'll teach you how to live, how to be the strongest. We'll kill your enemies! We'll protect you with our blood."

"All you need is me — I'm ecstasy. Nothing else matters. Take me and I'll take you away."

"You're not leaving this house, Maria! I hate your friends! I hate your clothes! And I'm not letting you leave here again."

"Take me, Maria. I'll take you away so quickly. I'll give you relief. I'll end all your cares. Take me, Maria. It's so easy, so fast, so painless."

"Please, Maria, come with us. We're your sisters. We can help you."

The actors were placed in a semicircle around her. The voices grew louder while Maria closed her eyes.

"You're a slut."

"Take me, I'm painless."

"We'll protect you with our blood."

The father made hitting noises with his fists. The drugs whispered in her ear. And the pressure to join the gang would have been enough to make me succumb. Stacy motioned to raise the voices and spun Maria in a circle. On the fourth turn, Maria dropped to her knees and let out a guttural cry as she reached for the sisters.

One sister came over and held her. "We love you, Maria. Please come home."

The girls sat on the floor crying in each others' arms while the interns canvassed the room to make sure everyone was all right. Liz nudged me to see if I was okay. I nodded and looked around the room for Patty. She had walked out of the session a few minutes after it started and hadn't returned.

The adolescents took their seats, and Stacy spent the next thirty minutes processing the drama. She asked if Maria's situation brought up similar memories or feelings. A nine-year-old boy spoke of his drug overdoses and suicide attempts. A ten-year-old cried as he shared that he had been sodomized by his father. My chest went numb when I heard the boy speak, and if it wouldn't have drawn attention to me, I would have stood up and left the room.

Friday's morning meditation was on abandonment. I tensed when I heard the word. I had been in constant pain since Anne left, but I wasn't sure if it was because I felt abandoned by her... or temporarily set aside.

The meditation came around to me.

"I pass." They all looked at me. I hadn't said anything about Anne in group since my first day in the program and Liz looked as if she was ready to call me out. I stared back at her. "I said, I pass."

She let it go.

The afternoon group met on the lawn. Liz, Patty and I grabbed a cup of coffee and stayed behind on the couch.

"What is the deal with your therapist?" Liz asked. "You look like you've been jilted by a lover." I tried to explain the relationship, but what happened between Anne and me didn't seem to translate.

"Was this a sexual relationship?" Liz asked.

"No. But my love for her is so strong it sure makes me question my sexuality." I looked at Patty. "Are you sure I'm not gay?"

"Are you sexually attracted to women?"

"No. But the idea doesn't repulse me either. And to tell the truth, I'm so hungry to be nurtured, I'd have sex with a woman just to be held."

Patty hit me across the knee. "Don't do that."

"Why not?"

"Well, first of all, you don't want to mislead a well-intended lesbian just because you want to be held, and secondly, being nurtured shouldn't cost you anything. Sex for affection is what your father taught you, and there are other ways to find the comfort you need."

"Patty, I'm a grown woman. What am I supposed to do? Walk up to somebody and say, 'Excuse me, I have the emotional mentality of a five-year-old, could you please hold me?'"

"It's better than saying, 'If you hold me, I'll give you sex.' " She shook her head. "At some point in your life, you're going to have to have more respect for your body than that."

I reached down and lifted up her self-defiled arm.

"Yes, we should have more respect for our bodies than that."

She grinned. "Funny how we tell each other what we need to hear."

"Yes, funny."

Liz put down her coffee. "I don't understand," she said. "Did this therapist fall in love with you?"

"I don't know exactly how she feels about me. I only know that she loves me."

"Is she married?" Patty asked.

"Yes, but she didn't leave with her husband."

They looked at each other and started to laugh. "Dawn, somebody wouldn't have to be gay to be attracted to you." Liz said.

"If she was attracted to me, she hid it well. I never sensed it was sexual."

"Sounds like she's running from you," Patty said.

Running from me? I wanted to believe it, but it didn't feel true.

"No, she's not running from me. She's out looking for herself."

On Tuesday mornings, our group joined a group of the inpatients for a session that was held in the family room of the main building. We sat around a fireplace as the doctor of psychology running the discussion gave us a lengthy title to describe her position. I decided to dislike her immediately. Even before I noticed she was as old as my mother, as proper as an English teacher, and she sat up in her chair like one of those plastic dolls that only bent at the waist, her butt cheeks so taut she looked as though she was going to tip over on her head.

"Hello, ladies, my name is Dr. Wesley and I would like to welcome you to the women's group. In this session I want you to be free to speak your mind about any issue that you might not want to discuss in front of a man." At the time, there were no men in the outpatient program, so it didn't make much difference to our group.

"Ladies, would anybody here like to bring up an issue?"

After several minutes of silence, Liz spoke up. "Before I started therapy, I thought I was special. I could do anything that I set my mind to. It was like I was magic. But now, it's gone. My doctor told me the magic wasn't real, it was just a part of my ego defenses."

"Let me try to explain that," Dr. Wesley said. "A part of a child's developmental psychology includes a stage of egocentrism. In that stage, the child believes that everything revolves around them. They can manipulate their surroundings to be whatever they desire. It sounds like you may have become arrested at that level of emotional immaturity and you now need to recognize that you have limitations."

Liz looked like she was dying and the doctor looked like she believed the world revolved around her. "Excuse me," I said, "but Liz came out of a slum in Texas to become a senior executive for a major corporation. That is magic. She manipulated her surroundings to get what she desired."

"If that is the case, then Liz is a talented woman, but children who were abused often wish to feel exceptional. For a doctor or therapist to encourage that belief is to infantilize them."

Infantilize them? "So if you think you're special, you're sick?"

"Excuse me, but I don't think I know your name."

"Dawn."

"Well, Dawn, children from dysfunctional families often develop ego defenses that make them feel superior to others."

I turned to Liz. "But Liz isn't talking about being superior to others, she's talking about being special. And she is. The only difference now is that somebody with some perceived authority told her she wasn't, and she believed him."

"I'm sure Liz's doctor knows how to handle her case."

"It doesn't sound like help to me."

I was looking for a fight. She wouldn't indulge me.

When the session was over, Stacy walked me back to our group. She had been there taking notes in the back of the room. We strolled through the eucalyptus trees back to the other side of the hospital. We had developed a quiet rapport. I hadn't given her any trouble, and it felt as though she was starting to like me.

"Dawn, I think the specialness Dr. Wesley was trying to explain was the grandiose illusion of the ego, when people feel they are more powerful, beautiful, or more intelligent than others. They find people who will feed the illusion that they are indeed the best. The specialness that I think you were touching on is not called grandiosity, it's referred to as grandeur."

"What's the difference?"

"Grandeur is the real power and beauty of our souls. It's the essence of our being. The talents and creativity that make us uniquely different and equally special."

"How can you tell one from the other?"

"A grandiose personality will be blown over by the first sign of criticism or imperfection. Underneath are deep feelings of shame and worthlessness that the ego is trying to hide from."

That would explain my ego. "But the grandeur of the soul," she said, "is as solid as a rock. It can never be destroyed."

"Then it's my ego that makes me want to hit that doctor."

"Your defensiveness in group may have been your ego trying to protect your pride. When you find yourself, you won't need to do that anymore."

When I found myself, I wouldn't need to do a lot of things.

The following Monday, I had my weekly appointment with Dr. Smith. It was our third session together, and each one was more frustrating than the last. I knew I needed his help, but at the same time, I didn't want to need him at all. In our sessions, the conflict I had with him made my skin crawl and the frustration drove me to tears. Neither of us understood my reaction. While it intrigued him, I was just glad our sessions were brief.

That evening, I picked up some fast food, handed it to Phil and went up and crawled in bed. At 3:00 a.m., I was awakened by a light pouring into the room. A full, harvest moon framed in the arch of my bedroom window.

He will help you.

The message came with a vision of Dr. Smith, his short-trimmed beard setting off his long, black eyelashes and sea-green eyes.

The following day, I was sitting in a group about nutrition. I found the lecture elementary, so I rested my head in my hand and began to doze off. A moment later, a distinct photo of a naked child suddenly appeared in my mind, and I was struck with a wave of nausea. My knees began to tremble as I stood up and walked outside for some fresh air.

I sat down on the lawn and rubbed my eyes. My body was having hot flashes, as if I had a sudden case of the flu, while my mind flashed abstract images of a naked girl lying flat on a beige-carpeted floor. The fear that I was about to die poured through every cell in my body. *I don't want to know this. I'll die if I know this.*

I stood up and walked into the cafeteria for a drink. It was an hour before lunch and the only two people in the commons were a nurse and Dr. Smith. I went up and told him what was happening. He looked down at my trembling hands.

"My 11:00 appointment just canceled," he said. "Let's see if we can find a room to talk."

He walked me into a small conference room. I sat down on the couch while he took the chair.

"What's going on?"

"It feels like a memory."

"How are you most comfortable retrieving your memories?"

"Anne would have me close my eyes and go down a staircase. At the bottom I opened a door."

"Is that what you want to do?"

"I guess."

"Okay, then close your eyes and picture yourself at the top of a staircase. When you reach the bottom, I would like you to open the door and tell me what you see."

I pictured the same spiral staircase that I had in the past. As I walked down the steps, all I could see in my mind was thick gray fog.

"It's very foggy," I said. "It's early in the morning. I can barely see where I am." I felt the cold dampness of the early morning fog that often rolled into La Jolla. "I'm in the car with my dad. We're at a park."

"How old are you?"

"I'm six. There are two men in the fog... no, they're in the window. They're watching me with my dad."

"Do you know the men?"

"Yes, Mr. Thomas and Mr. Unger; they're my dad's friends. I'm afraid they're going to come in. My dad tells me I'm safe... he's protecting me."

My voice started to crack. "I feel my dad's protection. I feel the strength of his body... but... but he's the one who brought me here." Tears streamed down my checks.

"Don't leave, Dad. Please don't leave."

"What's happening, Dawn?"

My eyes opened and I stared at the floor. "He said he was going to walk down the hill to have a cigarette. When he got out of the car, Mr. Unger came in."

The picture of the naked child was now branded on my mind. She looked to be about ten-years-old, her skin fair and her body long and skinny like mine. Long, brownish-blonde hair fell limp around her soft round face. Her eyes were closed, and her small, bluish lips curved down toward a red blood-stained slit that ran around the center of her neck. "When Mr. Unger was through with me, he showed me a picture. A Polaroid picture of a dead girl lying on the floor. He said he was my friend and he wanted to protect me. He told me bad things happen when little girls talk, and he didn't want to see anything bad happen to me."

I rested my head in my hands. "I knew I was never supposed to remember this. These men are going to kill me. They're going to kill me!" I felt as if my life was over. I pulled my knees to my chest and curled up into a ball.

"No, they're not. They can't hurt that little girl anymore. You grew up, and you're safe."

"No, I'm not! I'm not safe anywhere!"

He handed me some tissue as I lifted my head and took some deep breaths.

"How could he share me with his friends?" I cried. "How could he give me away?"

"I'm sorry."

I felt like a naked child in front of three grown men, the shame covering me like indelible ink.

"Is this real? Did this really happen to me?"

"It looks real to me. I'm not sure if the fog you describe was part of the memory, or if your mind wasn't ready to see it clearly. But I believe it happened."

"How? How could I forget this?"

"If children can't remove themselves from danger, their minds do it for them."

"But I loved my dad. Wouldn't I have hated him for doing this to me?"

"We need our parents' love to survive. That's why kids blame themselves for abuse."

I picked up a pillow and held it against my chest. "Could anything else be causing this? A brain tumor, a nightmare, anything?"

"I'm sorry, Dawn. There is no other phenomena to explain what you've been experiencing."

I stared at him, shaking my head in disbelief.

"Dawn, I can't tell you what all happened to you as a child, but in order to heal from this ordeal you're going to have to trust your feelings."

"How can I trust my feelings when I've been betrayed by my own memory?"

"Your memory didn't betray you. It protected you."

I wanted to die. When it was just my father, I could hold on to the belief that I was special. That in his own demented way he loved me. But this memory shattered everything I had left. The degradation felt so deep, I didn't ever want to be seen again.

Dr. Smith stayed with me for the hour, then walked me back to my group. On the path back, I noticed my body. It felt like a metal bar had been removed from my lower spine. I had more flexibility, stood taller, and was at peace with Dr. Smith.

In the afternoon group, I described the new memories, doubting the experience but remembering details. Mr. Unger was a molester. Mr. Thomas was a voyeur. I could see his face in the window. I could remember my skin pressed against the cold vinyl seats.

The group participated in my process, except for our youngest member, Denise. She sat in the corner sucking on her cigarette, preoccupied with a note. She asked to leave before the end of the session and as she walked out the door she threw me a folded piece of paper, a poem she had written during our group.

When she left, I read it.

Dawn's Game

Tattered webs of veiled memory
parted by digging fingers
probing into darkened scaled closets
grab the handle-peek inside!
Quench the thirst of questioning
so strong—so strong
to crack from revelations
an undying need to know
to turn the corner
never ending search for sanity's sweet calling
and what is it worth
nothing
that's the game
you got your answer
_____ do you feel?

I filled in the blank in my mind so I could finally hear it in my soul. <u>How</u> do you feel? I didn't know the answer, but I was ready to hear the question.

I came home that night and called my sister. The two men were friends of our family. Thomas had been an architect. Unger had been a pharmacist. My sister remembered them well and didn't have any problem believing the memory. She told me Mr. Unger was in jail. He had been caught a couple of years ago running the largest steroid ring in the South. It was a sick kind of validation, the kind that made me want to hang up and crawl into bed, hoping that a long nights sleep would make it all go away.

In the morning I woke up enraged, and ran to the beach to try and calm myself down. I ran four miles and I still had the desire to kill. I came back to the garage and hit a heavy bag with a baseball bat. When the bat broke, I threw it into the garage door and called Karen.

"I'm not going to the hospital today," I said.

"What's going on?"

I told her about the new memories and she asked me to come in to her office. An hour later, I blasted through her door.

"Where the fuck is Anne?" I yelled.

She looked up from her blue-cloth chair. "Why is that important to you right now?"

"Because I need her!" I grabbed a pillow and threw it onto the couch. "I have to tell her about the memories. Damn it! Why isn't she here?"

The pain tore through the anger, and I doubled over in tears.

"I need her. I need her to hold me."

Karen got up and sat next to me on the couch. "Dawn, don't you think this is what you felt like when you were a child? You had just been molested by your father and his friends, and you wanted to have a mother you could come home to—a mother who would understand your pain and hold you in her arms."

"But I don't want my mom to hold me. I want Anne to."

"Anne isn't here, but if you need to be held, I'll hold you."

I stood up and walked across the room.

"Dawn, I know you want Anne right now. But the intensity of the emotions you're dealing with isn't just about Anne. It's about all the experiences in your life that have been similar and never expressed. It's called transference phenomenon."

"Transference phenomenon?" There's a name for this?

"Repressed feelings like you are experiencing often come out in the therapeutic relationship."

"So my feelings about Anne are really about my parents?"

"I think that many of them are."

I shook my head. "I've been in therapy for a year. Why am I just now hearing about this?"

"I've been trying to get you to look at the similar feelings you have for Anne and your father for months."

"Yes, but you never told me why."

"It's the therapist's responsibility to pick up on the transferences, not the client's."

"That's ridiculous. Anne couldn't read my mind. And neither can you."

"You're right, but would it have made a difference if you had known?"

"Yes. It would have helped me understand why my emotions have been killing me."

"Dawn, up to the time Anne left, you hadn't been showing any emotion."

"That doesn't mean I haven't been having any." I turned around and hit the wall. "I hate this relationship."

"Our relationship?"

"The therapeutic relationship."

"Why do you hate it?"

"It's unfair, unbalanced, and it threatens my dignity!"

"Like being molested by adults?"

"If that's a transference, then yes. Therapy to me is like being molested by adults. You have the power and I get screwed."

Karen handed me a tissue and sat back in her chair. I walked over to the couch and slid down in my seat. "What a waste of time," I said.

"What's been a waste of time?"

"Therapy. I was very careful about the feelings I shared with Anne. I was ashamed of the thoughts I believed were neurotic or irrational so I kept them to myself. If I had known those feelings had more to do with my childhood than they did with Anne, I would have been freer to explore them."

"Anne's a therapist. She would have seen your feelings as transferences, not as irrational or neurotic."

"Yes, but I didn't know that, and I didn't know she knew that."

"But she was your therapist. You were supposed to be talking to her about what you thought were irrational thoughts."

I shook my head. "You don't understand. I needed Anne. I needed her to love and care about me. I wanted her to like me as a person, not see me as some whining, irrational pain-in-the-ass."

"What was the fear of showing her all your feelings?"

"That she'd leave. That she wouldn't want to see me again."

"She did leave."

Tears streamed down my checks. "Yes, but that wasn't because of me."

"That's right. We can't control other people's actions by our behavior. You could have proved to Anne that you were the best client in the world and she still would have left."

I dropped my head in my hands. "God, how did I get so screwed up?"

"You're not screwed up. And I don't blame you for being angry about not knowing about transferences, but now is the time when it's important to stick with the process. I know this is painful, but we're going in the right direction."

I picked up my keys and got up to leave.

"I want you to go back to the hospital tomorrow. I'm going to call Stacy to have her set up your psychodrama."

"What do you want me to do a psychodrama on?"

"Leave that to Stacy. It's time you let some other people take care of you."

I came home and lay down on my bed. The anger I was feeling toward Anne felt like such a betrayal of the love. But was it really love? Or just transference?

The next day, our group entered the psychodrama building. I sat between Patty and Liz while the adolescence unit entered the room. I recognized most of the kids from the week before. Stacy gave a brief introduction and asked me to enter the circle. With her arm around my shoulder, we walked around the room, my stomach churning as if I had to perform the lead in an elementary school play.

"Dawn, can you tell the group a little bit about yourself?"

"I'm 33 years old, married, and I have three children."

"How old are your children?"

"Samantha's six, Michael is three, and Erica just turned two."

"Sounds like a busy family. Can you tell us why you are in the partial program?"

I hated saying the word. "Incest. I was sexually abused by my father and some of his friends."

"Does any particular memory come up for you that you would like to deal with today?"

I went with my first thought. "When I was five, my dad drove me into a canyon to punish me."

"How were you punished?"

"He raped me."

"Can you describe your father to the group? Tell us about his mannerisms and how you remember him that day." She rubbed my shoulders as we walked around the circle.

"He was gruff, his voice was low, angry."

"Could you pick out somebody in the room to play your father?" I scanned the room. My eyes landed on an older gentlemen who was about my father's age. It was unusual to see a man over 40 in the program. I pointed to him and he came to the center of the circle. The interns pulled out two chairs and arranged them side by side like the front seat of a car.

"Was your mother home at the time?"

"Yes. We were supposed to be going to the store. I didn't want to go with him but she said I had to."

"Could you pick out somebody to play your mother?" I chose Liz. She looked like my mother, dark with short brown hair. They were both in their 50s and had the same Southern drawl. I told Liz that my mother had a stubborn, condescending way of dealing with me. She made light of my concerns by laughing at me and supported my father as the benevolent dictator.

"Can you pick out some people to play your husband and your three children?"

I looked around the room and saw a Latino gang leader holding up his hand. He was as tall as Philip, so I called him up. He high-fived his friend and came to stand next to me. My children were easy to select. Samantha was played by an African-American girl. Obviously darker, but the gentle spark that radiated from her eyes felt similar to the light I saw in Samantha's. My son was played by the nine-year-old boy whose hair was as white as Michael's. I chose Denise, the teenager in my group, to play my youngest daughter, Erica. Denise stood up from her chair and paid me the ultimate compliment of taking off her sunglasses.

Stacy and several interns prepared for the scene, the interns standing behind the cast and instructing them what to say. They placed my father in one seat of the car and my mother standing outside of it. My children were in a huddle off to the side. The boy playing Philip stood waiting for his cue.

The scene started with the voice of my father: "Get in the car, Dawn, we're going to the store."

My mother stood in front of me. "Now, Dawn, it's time to go to the store with your father. Go on now, get in the car."

I stood up to play my part, and as soon I did, it didn't feel like a role. I felt as if I was five-year-old, frustrated beyond words, frightened to leave the house with my father, sensing that if I did I would somehow be terribly hurt.

"I don't want to go, Mom. I don't want to go."

"Dawn, get in the car. If your dad wants you to go with him, you go with him. He's the boss of this family and we do what he says."

I lost awareness of the room. My vocabulary was reduced to a child's.

"I don't want to go!"

"As long as you're under our roof, you'll do what we say. Now get in the car!"

"Shut up, Mom! Shut up!"

"Don't you talk to me that way, I'm your mother!"

"You're so stupid! Stupid! Stupid!" I clenched my fist.

"Don't constrict your anger," Stacy said, "tell her everything you wanted to say." Two staff members came over and held a pillow between Liz and me.

"Hit the pillow," Stacy said.

"Dawn, your father's waiting. Get in the car."

"Can't you see what he's doing to me? Can't you?"

"You're going with him, Dawn. Get in the car." I began to hit the pillow. The force of my punches was pulling my feet off the ground.

"No. Stop him! Don't make me go! He going to hurt me, Mom, he's going to hurt me."

"Dawn, that's nonsense. Your father would never hurt you."

"Get in this car," my father said.

"No. Please, no. I don't want to go. Please... please."

"We're your parents. We know what's best for you, and you'll do what we say."

"Get in this car," said the raised voice of my father.

"I hate you, Mom! I hate you!"

She laughed at me. "Dawn, you're just going to the store. Now get in the car."

"I hate you forever and ever," I cried.

I sat in the seat next to my father. He slid next to me and put his hand on my thigh. I jumped out of my seat and danced around frantically.

"Don't touch me! Don't touch me!" I lurched toward my mother. The two therapists held me back.

"Hit the pillow."

I yanked my arm from their embrace and hit the pillow with a vengeance. Liz stayed in character, badgering me till my knees buckled and I started to sob.

"Mom." The young African-American woman's voice softly rose from the side of the room.

"It's Samantha, Mom. I'm here and I need you."

I went from a five-year-old to a helpless mother.

"I'm so sorry, Samantha. I'm so sorry I left you with him. I didn't know. I didn't know what happened to me. I'm so sorry."

The girl playing Samantha stepped forward. "I love you, Mom. I need you to help me grow up. Please, Mom, please come home where you belong."

The Latino boy playing Philip came up and softly wiped my tears. "It's over," he said. "I love you. I'm here to protect you, and nobody can hurt you again."

I broke down in his arms. The adolescents playing my children came up and embraced me.

"We love you, Mom. Please come home."

The day after my psychodrama my anger toward my mother dissipated. But when I thought about Anne, feelings of betrayal and abandonment raged through my body.

On Friday, I left the group early and went to the library. I searched the computer for literature on the therapeutic relationship and a title caught my eye. *Banished Knowledge: Facing Childhood Injuries*, by Alice Miller, M.D. Alice Miller was a psychiatrist. I assumed she was well known because I had heard of her. I picked out the book and read through the table of contents. The second section was entitled "My Path to Myself" and it explained how Dr. Miller used the transferences with her therapist to heal from her childhood wounds.

It is rare for the patient to perceive and feel the misery of his childhood by way of direct memories. Their memories are either completely banished, a prey to amnesia, or separated from feelings, emotionally inaccessible, and hence of little help. But the real history is betrayed by the behavior of the patient toward current reference persons, even toward those of secondary significance.

In the book, Dr. Miller suggests sharing the knowledge of the transference phenomenon with the patient to balance the therapeutic relationship and empower the patient with the use of the tool.

In this process the therapist need not even be the main object of the transference, for he is not alone in controlling the work, as he would be in analysis. The patient's increasing autonomy enables him, thanks to the tools he has been given, to supervise and resolve his transferences. He is capable at any time of taking up the emerging feelings with the current reference person, of confronting him inwardly, of challenging him, and of communicating his needs to him. He can use his transferred feelings to deepen his self-recognition, and he need not be ashamed of them.

I checked out the book and read through it that night. If I was ever going to see my soul in Anne's, I figured I'd have to go through the transference's first.

In the morning, I called Karen.

"Karen, does it make any difference if I'm angry at my mom or angry at Anne?"

"No... I don't think so. The important aspect about the transference is to recognize the perception and allow the feelings. I don't think it matters what face you attach to it."

"Good, because I think that's part of what my relationship with Anne is all about. Every time I think of her, I access emotions I didn't know I had."

"Does this mean you're ready to talk about the similarities between Anne and your father?"

"Yes, I'm ready."

Chapter 8

It was my last week at the hospital, and I felt like a different person. Not necessarily better, just different — almost hollow.

The security of our group would have been difficult to leave except that a new patient had been admitted on Friday and by Monday the dynamic of the group had changed. What had once been a safe place was now a battleground. Liz and I were losing our turf to a preppy-looking thirty-year-old who had all the answers and none of the problems.

Her name was Kathy. By her second day in the group, she had mentioned her master's degree in psychology 37 times. Her response on a trust issue was buried somewhere in a lengthy description of a lesson she taught to a Sunday school class, and if she told me what sorority she was an alumna of one more time, I would have been ready to knock her out.

By Wednesday, I couldn't stand to sit with her through another group. I went to the hospital early and caught Stacy before our session. We walked into her office, and she offered me a seat.

"What's going on?" she asked.

"This new woman, Kathy. She's driving me crazy. I can't stand to be in the same room with her."

Stacy got up and shut the door.

"Is this a transference or something?" I asked.

"Transferences are when you transfer your feelings from one person onto another. For example, if you had unresolved emotions with your first husband, you might transfer those emotions onto your second husband. I don't think that's what's happening here."

"Then what is happening?"

"What causes a situation like what you are experiencing with Kathy is called projection."

"What's a projection?"

"Projection is when we project personality traits of our own onto other people."

"You mean this obnoxious, controlling woman is trying to show me something about myself?"

"I think so. You see, the people you have connected with in the room reflect a part of yourself you like. You have bonded through mutual, likable traits. The people in our lives like Kathy, whom we dislike or even hate, tend to show us parts of ourselves we don't want to acknowledge."

"Are you sure about that?"

"Dawn, if she wasn't amplifying a part of you that you dislike, she wouldn't be able to upset your peace of mind to the extent that she has."

"How do I find out what the projection is?"

"Write down what you find annoying about her. Then put it in the first person."

I went back to the group. It seemed to me that Kathy's input was calculated. Her responses told us little about the way she felt and instead were centered on how she wanted us to think of her as a person. I wrote on my note pad.

She's trying to control what we think of her.

I put the sentence in the first person.

I try to control what people think of me.

My muscles released. My stomach sank . Ouch, that hurts. After the session, I went back to Stacey's office.

"That was a humbling experience," I said.

"What's that?"

"I often base what I'm going to say on what I want other people to think of me. I try to prove that I'm intelligent or accomplished, instead of just being who I am."

Stacy nodded and asked me to sit down. "When you're trying to prove yourself, what is it you're looking for?"

"I guess I'm looking for acceptance."

"So when Kathy is trying to impress the group by her accomplishments or perceived skills, what is she really looking for?"

"Acceptance." My eyes welled as my shoulders sunk in toward my body.

"When children grow up in an environment that is either too controlling, or at times out of control, they're not able to fully secure an identity. If we don't develop a strong sense of self, we become hungry for acceptance from others."

A tear rolled down my cheek. Stacy stood up and handed me a box of tissues.

"Dawn, Kathy wants people to see her the way she wants to see herself. I admit she's doing a song and dance in group, but it comes from a painful need."

"Please tell me my song and dance doesn't look as bad as hers."

"It depends who's watching it. Kathy looks different to every person in that room, and so do you. That's the point. You can't control what people think of you. And even if you could, it wouldn't solve the problem."

"And the problem is what I think of myself?"

"Yes, and the thoughts about ourselves are really the only thoughts we can control."

I stood up slowly and wiped my eyes.

"Dawn, you already are all the things you try to be, and if you can acknowledge your strengths and become secure with your identity you won't struggle to have them secured by others."

"I don't even have an identity any more."

She smiled. "You do, but before we can find what's real, we have to eliminate what isn't."

I returned to group the following morning. Kathy entered the room a few minutes later. I sat through the day without irritation. She was free to play her song and dance. I was free not to.

On my last day in the hospital I said my good-bye's to the group and went to the lobby to meet Dr. Smith. As I took a seat, a newsmagazine on the top of the coffee table caught my eye. *The God Particle* was a feature article, a report about modern physics. I thumbed through the pages and found the story. In the article, a scientist described God as a black hole in space that emanated light particles into the universe that created the world we see. The image the description brought to my mind was soothing. God as a black hole in space seems far less threatening than an old, angry, white guy sitting on a throne until Judgment Day.

"Sorry, I'm late," Dr. Smith said.

"That's okay, it gave me time to find something I might be interested in."

I put the magazine in my purse and followed him into a conference room. It was an easy session. He signed my release form, and I thanked him for his service. When we parted, he reached out his hand.

"Would you accept a hug?" I asked.

"No, I can't," he said. "Therapeutic ethics."

I smiled. "Someday I'm going to have to read that chapter."

I shook his hand and walked back to Stacey's office. One more signature and I would be free.

Stacy smiled when I walked in the door, moved some books off her chair and asked me to sit down.

"Do you feel any better than when you started the program?"

"I feel very different from when I started."

"I haven't heard you say much about your therapist. You still having problems with her?"

"Yes, but now that I know about transferences, I think I can deal with it better."

She handed me the paper work. "Then you understand how transferences and projections can get in the way of the truth?"

"Yes, and if it wasn't for a card she gave me before she left, I would probably think the whole relationship was based on my transferences."

She looked at me like I still believed in Santa Claus. "Dawn, therapists are like parents. We want them to love us, accept us, and at times we want to believe that we are the most important people in their lives. When you're in that state of mind, you can read a million things into a card that do not really exist."

I signed the papers and left. Was I really so delusional I couldn't read a simple card? Or was separating my truth from other people's opinions one of the hardest challenges of my life?

I came home from the hospital and picked up the mail. On the top of the pile was a postcard from Anne. It was simple. There wasn't much I could read into it.

Hi Dawn,

Enjoying life on a tiny island in South Thailand. Front of postcard shows our bungalows—very quiet, beautiful. Warm water, good snorkeling, weather perfect. Am trying to make plans to go to Australia in December and may not return until January.
Think of you and really hope you're doing well.

Love,
Anne

March popped into my mind as I read the word January. It was a relief. She wouldn't be contacting me until March, which would give me more time to work through my feelings and better understand the different levels of our relationship.

I took the postcard up to the nest and put it in the file with Anne's picture. There was no need for another reminder of her around my house. My feelings of loss were constant, my longings for her unabated.

Christmas came and went, taking every ounce of my energy to make it a happy occasion for my children. I would have been kidding myself if I had thought I pulled it off. All the Power Ranger and Barney dolls in the world were not going to change what was happening to their mom or bring back the family members who had now disappeared.

I continued to see Karen. Through my transferences with Anne, abuse memories blistered to the surface like a bad case of chickenpox. Memories of my seventh year were coming back into my awareness when my symptoms began to worsen and Karen went on a two-week vacation. She referred me to Judith while she was gone, a therapist in the suite who had recently moved into Anne's old office. I wanted to meet her. Anne and Karen had both told me about Judith's expertise in the technique of guided imagery. She taught on the subject throughout the country and the clients in her private practice were mostly psychologists and therapists.

The week Karen left, Judith and I made an appointment. It was a rainy winter day. Judith walked out of her office just as I entered the lobby, and when our eyes met, a bolt of thunder rattled the building. The fluke was so eerie we just stared at each other.

"Do you always introduce yourself with thunder?" I asked.

She laughed. "I was about to ask you the same thing."

We joked on the way back to her office, both of us trying to shake off the coincidence.

Anne's old office looked different. The dent in the wall I had made when I threw the doorstop was now hidden by a neoclassical loveseat. Across from the couch and facing each other were two overstuffed tapestry-upholstered chairs.

Judith had the same classic look as her office. She was a tall, slender woman in her late 40's with fine, China-doll skin and thick, black hair that curled to her shoulders, her black silk suit and white scoop-neck blouse flowed with the sleek lines of her body. She asked me to be seated while she left the room to check in with an intern. I walked over to an antique hutch that encased her books. Traditional psychology, medical journals, biology and physics were the subjects of the books I glimpsed.

Judith came back into the room, closing notebooks, pushing mail out of the way and talking, articulate but non-stop.

"Have a seat," she said.

She calmed when we sat down and made eye contact; her energy was focused on me, and I connected with it.

"Karen told me you've been dealing with repressed memories," she said.

I gave her my matter-of-fact rendition of the abuse. She absorbed more than listened. Her focus was wise, not intense. I felt safe with her. It was time to go further.

"Repressed memories seem to be only half of my problem," I said.

"What's the other half?"

"I think I'm receiving a calling."

"What kind of a calling?"

My stomach tightened and churned, the skeptical side of my mind was fighting every word — shooting me with pangs of humility as I tried to explain the unexplainable.

"I'm not sure exactly, but it feels like some kind of spiritual power is pulling me into service. Leading me down this path to-wards something I'm supposed to do."

"When did this start?"

"About a year and half ago, this comet of energy started whirling in my chest, sending signals throughout my body. I don't belong to any religion, and I don't have much of a concept of God, but by this very strong primordial instinct, I really think I'm receiving some sort of a calling."

I wanted to cry. My fear of God, and the shame that I wasn't worthy enough to know such a power, collided together the way waves do in a storm.

"Then, a few months after the energy started, I began to receive messages."

"Can you describe to me what you experience when you receive a message?"

"It's like a telepathic thought that enters my mind, but it's not being produced by my own thoughts. Sometimes these thoughts come spontaneously, and sometimes I have received them during guided imagery sessions."

She nodded.

"Does that sound strange to you?" I asked.

"No. We all receive messages — some people are just more tuned in to them than others. Do you get them often?"

"As often as I need them."

"Do they come with images?"

"Yes. In my mind, almost as if it comes from a world that arises from between my eyes, is an image of a very nurturing, strong and wise Indian looking woman who appears to be about my age. And more recently another much older looking woman appeared in a long, white cape with a high-pointed collar. She's majestic — like some sort of high priestess. I feel very humble in her presence"

"Do these women have names?

Names? "I don't know, Anne and I never asked. Is that important?"

"I don't know if it's important. It's just polite."

I started to laugh. "You want me to give these images a name?"

"No, I'm sure they already have them."

"They do?"

"Yes, the images you receive are the mind's way of communicating the different parts of our beings. If we ask for a name and interact with the image, we can find out more about it. Are the figures benevolent, strong, gentle, young, old, wise, masculine, feminine?"

"But do we have to go as far as to give them separate names?"

"It helps to distinguish them from other parts of the mind."

"You're making me feel like a multiple personality."

"We're all multiple personalities."

"We are?"

"Yes." She unwrapped a piece of candy and placed it in her mouth. "On one end of the spectrum is the person who loses consciousness as they go in and out of the different parts of their being. On the other end is someone like the Dali Lama who has brought all the different aspects of the mind into conscious awareness."

"Do you have other clients who receive messages from images?"

"Sure. That's what guided imagery is all about. Getting in touch with parts of you that you were not aware existed."

I felt a little stunned. It still surprised me when somebody older than me took me seriously.

"Do you know Anne Myers?" I asked.

"Yes, I do."

"I was her client for a year before she left. We became very close during that time, but since she left I've had a hard time figuring out what happened." I spent the next twenty minutes telling her about my relationship with Anne—the love I felt for her and the faith she had in me. I told her about the message I had received to let Anne go, the one about Mexico being the wrong direction, and the burst of energy in my head that told me when I saw Anne's soul, I would see my own. Then, I told her about the physical affection. The day Anne told me she was leaving and we held each other, surrounded by a feminine spirit that seemed to ignite something in me—a spark in the center of my being that now felt like a flame growing in my body.

And then I shared with Judith the feelings I had been too ashamed to share with any one, the painful longing for Anne that tore at me every day, torturing me as if I had been ripped from the womb prematurely.

"I've been very confused," I said. "Between my childhood yearnings, the transferences and the spiritual messages, I don't know what about our relationship was real."

"It sounds like you know exactly what was real."

"I do?"

"Yes. It sounds like there were transferences, counter transferences, and it sounds like it was a powerful relationship that allowed you to access a profoundly deep level of your mind."

"Then you think the message that when I see her soul I'll see my own was real."

"Yes, I do. I don't know how or when that will happen, but I believe it will."

Thank God. The first validation I'd had since Anne left.

"What's a counter transference?" I asked.

"Some of Anne's repressed emotions also could have been coming out in the relationship."

"You mean Anne's feelings for me might not have really been about me?"

"It happens. Therapists are people, too."

I sank back into the confusion.

"Tell me more about the symptoms you're experiencing," she said.

"I keep getting flashbacks of a construction trailer. And for the past month my hands have been cramping, like my circulation is being cut off."

"Do any feelings accompany the cramps?"

"I'm angry at Anne. I feel like she misused me."

"Did she?"

"I think I was hurt by her confusion, but I don't think Anne could have hurt me intentionally." I stared at the couch that covered my mark on the wall. "Then again, I didn't think my father could hurt me either." I swallowed the lump in my throat and told her I was ready to do a guided imagery.

"All right, but before we go into the flashback of the construction trailer you have been having, I want you to contact the two women you describe. Do you have a place where you meet them?" I told her about the image of the garden with the white bench under a lush tree that sat on a manicured lawn.

"Good, close your eyes and tell me when you're there."

That was it. No breathing, no music, no suggestions to relax.

"Tell me when you're in the garden and who you're with." I missed Anne's voice. I wasn't sure if I could access the images without the safety of Anne in the room, but within a minute the garden appeared and so did the two women.

"Okay, they're here."

"Ask them their names."

In my mind, I asked each one their name. And when I did, I telepathically received an answer. "The Indian woman's name is Elisa, and the older woman would like to be called Madame."

"Do either one of the women have anything they want to tell you today?"

I asked the question and waited for the response.

"Elisa told me to *trust myself.* Madame told me to *start writing.*"

"Start writing. Do you know what that means?"

"Yes, I do."

"All right, then. When you're finished with Elisa and Madame, I want you to thank them for coming and then leave the garden. And when you're out of the garden, I want you to go to the construction trailer and tell me what you see, sense or feel." I left the garden and suddenly, I began to smell coffee, peppermint gum, and the burning scent of rubber from the electric eraser that I used to play with on my dad's drafting board.

"Where are you?" Judith asked.

"I'm in a trailer with my dad and another man." The picture was vivid. "I'm sitting on a cabinet, naked. My hands are tied behind by back. My dad's sitting behind a drafting board and this man is standing in front of me."

"Do you know the man?"

"No. They're laughing at me — it's a game to them."

"Are you laughing?"

"No, my hands hurt from the cord they tied me up with. I hate this game. I want to go home."

"If you need help with the memories, you can bring in Elisa or Madame."

"No. Judith, I don't want to remember any more."

She took me through a series of suggestions to help me release the trauma. When I was finished, she asked me to bring my awareness back to the room. I opened my eyes. I felt like I had just endured my tenth round of chemotherapy.

"I don't know how much more of this I can take." I grabbed a tissue. "Judith, my dad seemed like such a normal guy. He helped me through college, bought me my first car. He was a hard worker, a successful businessman. He taught me many positive things. How could this action be coming from the same person?"

"Human beings are capable of being both bad and good. That your father had a very dark side doesn't mean he was entirely bad. His good qualities are still good."

I shook my head. "I don't want to believe this."

"Do you remember what Elisa told you before you entered the trailer?"

I looked at her. "Trust myself?"

"Yes."

"Do you believe this happened?"

"I believe something like this happened, but memory isn't perfect. One, or several events can collapse into one another. Time distortions can occur, and when the memory is dramatic and a child dissociates, the recall is often more abstract than a memory that was not repressed."

"If dissociated memory is abstract, then how can you tell what literally happened and which are images like the garden or the Indian women?"

"By your feelings. What is neurologically encoded in the body is the feelings of the experience. Whether those feelings arise with metaphoric images, or literal memory images, doesn't really matter. They rise to awareness because they are trying to communicate an event and give us a chance to heal from the experience."

"So, I can't always trust my memories?"

"You can always trust that your memories are trying to tell you something about your experiences and how you felt when you endured them. Dawn, if you didn't have the experiential base associated with the abuse you have recalled, you would not have had the reaction you had when Anne left. Highly functional people are not hospitalized when their therapist leaves unless there is a history of abandonment, betrayal, mistrust and every other emotion you have suffered. Those feelings came from somewhere, and every time you experience fragments of memory, whether every detail of it literally happened or not, you are healing from an experience that encoded those feelings in your body."

"Does that mean I'll never have perfect recall?"

"Total recall would revictimize you beyond what would be healthy. Trust your mind to give you what you need to heal and try to accept that you will probably never remember all the times, places, and details of what happened to you."

I didn't want to accept it. Reliving my childhood was like digging up a skeleton, and I wanted to see the body. Make it tangible — touch it, taste it, feel it like it was yesterday. I reached for my keys.

"Is this memory what you're supposed to write about?" asked Judith.

"No, I'm supposed to be writing a book, but I don't really know what it's about."

"Maybe it's about sexual abuse."

"No. I'm not writing about sexual abuse." I looked up at her bookshelf. "I've read a couple of articles lately about the evidence of God in the new findings of physics. Maybe I'm supposed to be writing about that."

"I have a book on the subject that you are welcomed to borrow."

"That would be great."

She scanned the shelf and took down the book. "But before you escape into physics," she said, "I think you should write about the abuse memory. You'll need to process it further."

"Okay."

She hugged me good-bye as if she had known me for months. I thought the thunder was a coincidence, but I knew from my comfort level with her that she was to be my next mentor.

I went home and wrote about the memories, piecing together feelings and flashbacks to try to get some idea of what had happened. When I had finished writing it all down, I was finally relieved of the intrusive thoughts about the construction trailer. And when I thought about Anne, all I felt was how much I missed her.

Philip came into the nest as I put away my journal. He had a towel around his neck and an unopened beer in each hand. I didn't like it when he drank, but at the same time I felt the alcohol somehow compensated for what I was unable to give him.

"Do you want to go up to the Jacuzzi?" he said.

"No thanks, I'm kind of tired."

He walked out like a rejected boy. It was breaking my heart to watch him suffer, but my body was tarnished by the touch of the molesters and even Philip's presence would bring on the repulsion.

In the morning, I awoke to his chest against my back. It was Saturday and the kids were still asleep.

"I'm lonely," he said as his hand caressed my thigh. "I don't want to pressure you, but I need to feel like you want me."

"I'm sorry. It's not that I don't want you... it's just that I can't be with you right now."

He turned me over on my back, his blue eyes fixed on mine. "I didn't do this to you, and I feel like I'm being blamed for it."

I couldn't answer. He dropped his head back on the pillow. "Then there's only one thing left for me to do," he said.

"What's that?"

"It's time to find a girlfriend." He jumped out of bed and put on his clothes.

"A girlfriend. You're really going to go find a girlfriend?"

"A man's got to do what a man's got to do."

He grabbed his keys off the nightstand. "I'll see you in a couple hours."

I lay back on my pillow, curious but not worried. Phil preferred fishing to a woman, even in his current condition.

At noon, his car pulled up and the kids and I walked out to greet him.

"Come on," he said as he grabbed my hand, "I want you to meet the new woman in my life." He opened the door to the van and an 18-month-old black Labrador retriever jumped out and licked me.

"They didn't have any females left at the pound, so she is really a he and his name is Maxx."

Maxx jumped all over me, as starved for affection as Phil was.

"So, Maxx, you're my new competition?"

Phil came up and hugged me. "Maxx and I will wait for you, as long as we have to."

The winter days were long, the nights often sleepless. My relationship with Karen was losing its energy. My transferences with Anne were as powerful as ever. I tried to talk to my friends about her, but my statute of limitations was running out and I was starting to get the same advice I would have given them: "She was your therapist, for God's sake. Get over it."

On the first of March, I felt more at ease. If my premonitions were correct, Anne would be home. She would call me, and then I'd know. Through her voice I'd be able to hear what was real and receive the clarity I needed to trust my love for her, and her love for me.

The month went by quickly. I had a seven-year-old birthday party for Samantha and her friends and before I knew it, it was the end of the month. Anne was home. I could feel it in my bones. But still, I hadn't heard from her.

I went up to the nest one afternoon and called Karen.

"Karen, I keep getting the feeling that Anne's back in town."

There was a long pause. "She was. I was waiting for our next appointment to tell you."

"What do you mean, 'was?'"

"She was home for a couple of weeks. She took off again a few days ago."

"What? Why didn't she call me?" I said.

"I don't know."

"Did she ask about me?"

Another long pause. "No. I'm sorry, she didn't."

Her answer knocked the breath out of me. "Do you know where she went or when she's coming back?"

"She moved. She packed up her stuff and took it somewhere up north. I think she was going to keep traveling."

"Karen, I went into the hospital the day she left. Doesn't she even want to know how I am?"

"I really think we need to talk about this in person. Why don't you come in for a session?"

"No, no... I need some time to think about this. I'll call you in a few days."

I hung up and floored myself in the nest.

How could she come back and not call? How could she come back and not even ask about me? Phil walked in and looked at me. Without a word, he took the kids out to dinner and then put them to bed.

I lay awake on the floor staring at the ceiling and breaking into sobs. The feeling of being shutout, left like an orphan by the one person who was finally supposed to love me, waved over me like a relentless sea. The pain that rose up into my chest from deep within my belly felt as old as time. Faces reel across my mind, the images of the people in my life whose love I depended on, who took it away when I needed it most. For the rest of the night, I rolled up in a blanket and sobbed until I couldn't breathe. When my stomach ached from the convulsions, my body completely exhausted from the tears, I lay back on the floor and watched through the window as a brilliant pink sky turned to a clear powder blue.

Love is not what you receive from others, it's what you have for them.

My heart warmed as the message entered my mind. In that still moment, lying alone on the cold floor, in a blanket soaked with my tears, I realized the love that I thought was dependent on others was something I already had. It was part of me that couldn't leave — the part of me I felt when I thought of the people I loved.

For the next few days I felt as though I had been released from prison. For the first time in my life I recognized love as my own experience, freed from the illusion that it only came from other people. I could survive by loving others, and as Samantha once tried to teach me, "the more you try to give love away, the more it comes right back at ya."

I walked into my next session with Karen and told her about my revelation.

"Dawn, if you now recognize that love is something that is within you, then what was it about your relationship with Anne that allowed you to feel it?"

"She was safe."

"Do you know why she was safe?"

"When I was in her arms, I didn't have to be on guard. I could just be who I am." I thought about the feelings she shared with me, and the note she gave me before she left. "I still can't believe she didn't ask about me."

"She's going through a divorce right now. I wouldn't take her actions personally."

"Is she all right?"

"She's fine. Anne knows how to take care of herself."

Karen picked up her pen. "Now that you know how you experience love, is it something you can begin to do with other people?"

"I have experienced love with other people — my kids, Phil, and my friends — but this experience with Anne is different."

"How?"

"I don't really know, but the love I feel for her is not fading away — it's getting stronger."

"I'm a little concerned about that. This relationship has too much power over you — it's beyond what's healthy."

"Believe me, I'm more concerned about it than you are."

"Do you think you're being obsessive?" she asked.

"Obsessive? I don't know. My feelings are powerful, but they're not frantic."

She wrote herself a note. "There are several reports out right now showing anti-depressants are an effective drug treatment for obsessions. You might want to consider it as an option. It could make your life more comfortable."

"I don't want to be more comfortable. I want to be better."

"Suit yourself, but I think it's time you start considering the possibility that you may not hear from Anne again."

"Why do you say that?"

"Dawn, I don't know where in your relationship it happened, but I think some emotional boundaries were crossed and that might be why you haven't heard from Anne."

"Why would that make her not contact me?"

"I'm sure Anne was aware of the transferences between you two. If she went out for counsel, which I think she did, just about anybody would have advised her to cut the relationship off."

"If she changed her mind about contacting me, why wouldn't she tell me?"

"I don't know, but I don't think you should expect to hear from her again."

The thought hurt too much. I checked out whether I needed to feel the pain.

"No. I'll hear from her again. Every instinct in my body tells me so."

"Okay, but you might want to ask yourself: Is it instinct, or denial?"

I didn't know the answer, but I knew I had to hang on to the hope.

Phil's love affair with Maxx looked much more rewarding than my love affair with Anne. Maxx and Phil ran on the beach, wrestled in the yard and rolled on the grass, chewing on each other's ears. I sat up in the nest and watched them out the window. They were both so present in their love for each other. Would I ever be so enlightened?

I wanted to contact Anne, but it didn't feel right, so I focused my energy on the book. The message to *tell the story* often came to me as I awoke in the early morning, but I had no idea what the story was, so I continued to look for one.

I searched for the meaning of the universe. Somewhere inside my pile of modern physics, psychology and philosophy books was a common thread that I was sure would lead to the answer. Einstein's quantum theory was over my head, but the challenge took me out of my misery. Or at least I thought it did until my mother called.

"Before I come up and see the kids again," she said, "I would like to talk to you about a few things."

"What do you have in mind?"

"Oprah Winfrey had a show on yesterday about false memories. Did you see it?"

"No, but I've heard about this before."

"Well, I think you should hear it again, because it's happening all over the country. These women on her show had been led in therapy to believe they had been sexually abused by their fathers."

"Mom, I've never been led in therapy, and if you're concerned that I have, why don't you and Dad come up and see my therapists?"

"The only person I want to talk to is Anne Myers."

It was a safe command. She knew Anne had been gone for months.

"This has nothing to do with Anne. I've had more memories released during session with other therapists than I ever had with Anne."

"She's the one who made the original diagnosis and, she's the only person I want to talk to."

"There was no diagnosis, and it's not possible to see Anne. You're welcome to come up and see Karen."

"Dawn, you and Anne Myers accused your father of abusing you and then she leaves the country. What kind of therapist is that? And where is she now? Where is she when I want to talk to her?"

"You had six months to talk to her between the time I told you about the memories and the time Anne left on vacation."

"Then when's she coming back?"

"She's not. She moved."

She started to laugh, and I started to cry.

"How do you know she didn't suggest your father abused you while you were under hypnosis?"

"I was never unconscious when we did guided imagery."

"You don't know that!"

"Yes, I do!" Why was I still on this phone?

She took a breath and reloaded. "If your father was hurting you, why would you go with him? Why would you let him do that to you?"

"I was a child. What else was I supposed to do?"

"You could have told me."

"I tried to. Remember the time in the bathroom?"

"That could have been a coincidence."

I cleared my throat so she wouldn't hear me crying. "I have to go."

"If you have all the answers, how do you explain the lie detector test your father took?"

"What lie detector test?"

"Your father went down several months ago and took one at the police department."

"Did he pass it?"

"Yes. I talked to a police officer and he said he did."

"Have you seen the test?"

"No."

"Do you know what questions were asked?"

"No, but your dad went down to the station and, the man said he passed it."

"Why don't you get the test and bring it up to show Karen and me?"

"No. I'm not going to do that. Your father said we have to be very careful about what we say or do. He thinks you might press charges."

I slammed down the phone.

My faith in humanity dissolved. My parents' protecting themselves against the legal system had become more important than feeling compassion for their own daughter.

I rifled through my desk for a number. I wanted the fast track now. The bullet cure. Something that would rid my body of the mounting resentment so I could get on with my life. I pulled up the card. Steve Rally was his name. A friend had recommended him a week ago and the name had stuck with me, not in my mind like a knowing, but in my chest where I was starting to feel what was true. It was time to call.

Steve called back in the morning and gave me his pitch about bioenergetics, a physical therapy designed to release trapped emotions in the body tissue.

"How long will it take?" I asked.

"That depends on you, and how hard you're willing to work."

"You all say that."

He asked me to come in and try it. I asked a few more questions and then clearly stated my position. "Steve, before you work with me, you should probably know, my definition of therapist is someone who is slightly less screwed up than I am."

He laughed, so I made the appointment.

I had one last session with Karen. She supported my decision to move on to a new healing modality, and we closed our relationship amiably.

The next day Steve came out to his lobby to greet me, a dark-haired man in his late thirties with big brown eyes and a full mouth that rested in a smile. His broad shoulders turned toward me.

"Hi, Dawn, I'm Steve." I stood while he shook my hand. He wasn't much taller than I was. I liked that.

"Come on back, I'll show you around." He took me into a soundproof room that turned out to be a large office equipped with bats, foam blocks, pillows and a body-length sparring cushion. I stared at the cushion.

"Can I beat you up?"

"Is that what you want to do?"

I smiled. If I had to be in the system, I was going to make it work for me.

"Yes," I said, "I want you to be the object of my resentment. And then, I want to beat the hell out of you."

He laughed. "Who do you resent?"

"Everybody."

"Do you want to sit down and talk about that?"

"No. I don't want to talk about it, and I don't want to be analyzed. I just want to beat the shit out of you."

He smiled and asked me to take off my shoes. "Stand in the middle of the room," he said. "Put your feet at shoulder width, slightly bend your knees and point your toes a little inward." I followed his instructions. "Now, bend over, drop your head between your shoulders and hold on to your ankles." I held the position. A few minutes later, my thighs shook from fatigue and a surge of anger poured up my legs and into my chest. I had the aggression of a line backer.

"How do you need to act out your anger?" he said.

"I need to push you." I stayed in the position. The anger continued to build while Steve held the body cushion in front of him and faced me in the middle of the room.

"Okay, let's go," he said.

I tore up from the floor, buried my shoulder in his sternum, and pushed him across the room. When we hit the wall, I threw him up against it until I heard the thud of his back smashing into the drywall.

"That was good," he said. "But this time I want to hear it."

Steve directed me back to the center of the room. I put my feet at shoulder width and grabbed my ankles. A minute, maybe two, and I had the rage of a killer. I stood up and pushed him. "You fuckin' bastard!" My mind regressed. He was my father's friends. As I pushed, screamed and listened to the thud of his back against the wall, most often he was Mr. Unger, the man who showed me the picture of the dead child. And after each time I tore up from the floor, I felt another layer of filth dissolved from my body.

For the next two months, I saw Steve twice a week. He would ask what I needed to do, and I would know. Even if it sounded strange, he followed my instincts. He leaned his chest against my body just so I could push him off. He pushed down on a pressure point in my pelvis that released a child's blood-curdling scream. If I cried, he cried with me. If I yelled, he yelled with me, and if I fought him, he let me win. Together we released more anger than I thought possible, stored in parts of my body I didn't know existed.

We worked together until I noticed a change in the anger I felt in my body. It wasn't stored aggression anymore, like heaps of molting lava attached to my intestines, it was a different kind of anger, like a hostile irritation from touching an infected wound.

More and more I thought about Judith. The pull in my chest was directing me to her. I had grown out of the teenage rebellious stage Karen handled well, and was ready for the deeper, broader knowledge Judith brought to her practice. Of course, I wasn't going to receive the kind of friendship I had with Karen. The edges to Judith's boundaries were clear and sharp, and I wasn't about to test them. She wasn't going to walk me to my car, or give me her home phone number, but then again, I no longer needed them. I closed my relationship with Steve and committed to weekly sessions with Judith.

I sat down across from Judith. She looked professionally stylish: wool pants with textured socks and a long low-necked red sweater that brightened her thick, black hair and fine, almost translucent olive skin. She slipped on a pair of small wire-rimmed glasses, the straight-edged top resting just under the ridge of her nose.

"You look better than the last time I saw you," she said as she confidently crossed her legs.

"I had more anger in my body than I thought was possible."

"I bet."

I leaned forward and heightened my attention. I knew from our last session that her questions were quick and unpredictable. To follow her train of though I would have to speed up my own.

"So what's coming up for you right now?" she said.

"Mostly the need for acceptance, and with that awareness comes a sense of insecurity."

"Acceptance for what?"

"For who I am. I want my parents to acknowledge the abuse and accept me for what I've been through and who I am because of it."

"What's your relationship with them like?"

"I don't talk to them anymore. My mom thinks I'm having false memories, and my dad has denied the abuse to everybody but me."

"That sounds painful."

"Yes, it is. The only way I could get back with my parents now is if I pretended the sexual abuse didn't happen." I looked up at the ceiling to catch a tear in my eye. "To tell you the truth, sometimes it hurts so bad that I consider it."

"People do recant their memories for just that reason."

"I know, but after I thought about it, I realized there really isn't any satisfaction in that type of acceptance."

She nodded. "Tell me more about the acceptance."

"I want them to acknowledge the abuse, the pain it has caused me and accept me for the person that I am — the person who endured the trauma."

"And do you?"

"Do I what?"

"Accept who you are. Your abuse, and the part of you that endured the trauma."

I felt I was on another road and not sure how I had gotten there. "I think I do, but it doesn't feel like it's enough. I still want acceptance from my parents."

"What if you never get it?"

"I don't know, but I probably never will."

"There's an old Buddhist teaching I've read about. Let me see if I can remember it correctly." She looked as though she was pulling it out of the air. "Oh yes...in your mind you must first kill your parents, then you shoot the Buddha."

"Shoot the Buddha?"

"Yes. If you continue to look for self-acceptance from a parent or a teacher, your sense of self is being based on somebody else's opinion. Your identity becomes vulnerable to the perceptions of others and that can make you feel very insecure."

"So if I had more acceptance for myself, I wouldn't need it from my parents?"

"That's the theory."

"I guess I don't have a choice anymore. I can't change my parents' mind."

"You never could."

I nodded and stared at the floor.

"How are you doing on your relationship with Anne?"

Oh...Anne. My body still tensed when I heard her name. My stomach constricted from the hunger. "I've had every emotion for her and its polar opposite, and there is still no waning of the feelings. She's on my mind every day." I looked up at Judith. "Do you think that's sick?"

"No. I believe that you loved Anne very much and that's going to take some time to get over."

"Do I have to get over it?"

"I can't answer that for you. That's up to you and what you're comfortable with."

Phil walked in the door a few minutes after I came home from Judith's office. In his hands was a case of beer, in his mouth a letter. A company on the East Coast had made an offer to buy ICON. We negotiated the offer for a week, then accepted a deal that put cash in the bank and freed us from the corporation.

Phil and I took the next week off. I arranged for one of my friends to watch the kids, and we boarded a flight to the big island of Hawaii. My anxiety washed away as we flew over the lava fields of Kona. What was happening in the minds of my parents no longer mattered. For the next week, I was going to nurture myself in the warm waters of the South Pacific.

Our first night on the island, a local waiter told us about a day hike — a trail that led to a remote, black, sandy beach on the east side of Wiapio. We packed some food and headed out the next morning, past the barren fields of lava that covered the western island, into the wet climate zone where the landscape changed from open fields to lush tropical forest.

We found the trailhead at the top of a 3,000-foot ridge. Below the cliff was the ocean, a vastness so inviting that for a moment I wanted to spread my wings and jump. Phil put on the backpack and, we began the hike down to the valley. A tropical shower intermittently broke through the sunshine and the 85-degree heat. In between the showers, we jumped into the waterfalls that cascaded into small pools that lined the path to the valley.

At the bottom of the grade, we turned down a narrow trail that took us through the jungle. Shaded by a grove of palm trees, we walked into the center of the valley where the long-eared leaves of philodendrons provided another layer of shade to the flowering red and blue impatiens that carpeted the valley floor. The air was fresh with the scent of the jungle. The beauty that surrounded us was magical.

Phil walked ahead while I stood on the trail, my body vibrating with the same subtle oscillation I used to feel at night. I thought of Anne. Wherever she was in the world, I wished her well. Then I picked up my pace and caught up with Philip.

When we reached the ocean we saw a few surfers. They had camped overnight, so we headed north to get even further away from civilization. The fifty-foot river that drained the jungle floor ran rapid where it entered the ocean. We walked up the stream to find a safer crossing. Phil held the backpack over his head while he waded across. Not as tall as he, I had to swim. He sat on the other side laughing.

"There's a snake!" he yelled. "No... it looks bigger than a snake!"

I knew he was kidding, but his words motivated me to swim fast.

We walked down the beach where our footprints were the only ones in the black sand. At the foot of the second ridge was a grassy knoll that perched over the beach. Two large palm trees shaded the grass. A hammock hung between them.

Phil and I looked at each other. We were in an oasis in paradise. We ran up the knoll and jumped into the hammock. Phil pulled out the leftover swordfish from our dinner the night before, drained the juice from a fresh pineapple, and we ate lunch. The rhythm of the ocean seemed to sway with the hammock. The food and the fresh air put me right to sleep.

An hour later, I awoke to a warm breeze blowing up my spine and a clear thought that brought me some peace. It was time to let go of my parents. The only acceptance I needed in this world was my own. If I was being true to myself, I could live in peace with my decisions, my circumstances, and my experiences.

Chapter 9

A small, colorful oriental vase sat on the shelf of the bay window in Judith's office. The background of the vase had a light green diamond pattern, in the forefront was a bold brink-red flower. The pot was another expression of Judith's eclectic, artistic flare — a side of her that was also reflected in the beaded African necklace she occasionally wore, and in the metaphors she sometimes used comparing an emotional state to the tempo of a classical concerto. Her intellectual persona kept our sessions interesting and gave me permission to ask the esoteric questions I might otherwise be reluctant to ask.

"Do you think we subconsciously attract, or create the things that happen to us in our lives?" I asked Judith during our next session.

"I think we subconsciously create re-abusive situations as adults to attempt to heal from childhood wounds, if that's what you're asking."

"But do you think we have the ability to create or choose what happens to us as children?"

"Dawn, you were not responsible for your father's actions."

"I realize I didn't create his actions, but maybe I came into this world feeling like I deserved to be treated that way."

I spent the next several minutes explaining the past-life images I had seen during guided imagery sessions with Anne, the images of the Chinese life where I lost my mother in the field. And the images of the life as a monk, where I misused other people, and at my death felt I needed to be punished for my sins.

"I think those thoughts carried forward into this life and had some effect on my sense of myself."

"I don't."

"You don't believe in reincarnation?"

"No. I don't"

"So you think we come into the world with a blank slate?"

"No. I think we come into the world with a personality disposition and with it a set of images or perceptions, but I believe those perceptions arose from the pool of the collective experiences of our humanity, not the process of one self in many bodies."

I imagined the cesspool of our humanity's collective experiences. It made me feel my life was a bubble coming up through pond scum.

"But several months later," I said, "after I remembered my father's abuse, I had a session where I saw the image of my past life as a monk, and my current life as a three-year-old child. I received the message that there was no need for punishment, that I had always been as innocent as a child."

"Sounds like a powerful message."

"It was, and it made me further believe that I lived a life as a monk."

"Maybe you did."

"So you do believe in reincarnation?"

"No. What I believe is that in guided imagery, the mind has an opportunity to communicate to us. Sometimes it communicates by memory, and sometimes by metaphor. And as we've talked about before, the truth behind the images is not necessarily in their literal interpretation as much as in the feelings the images convey."

"I'm confused."

"In the images you describe, the reality of your innocence was presented to you in a way that you could understand, a way that made it possible for you to correct your self-image. But I don't think you should take that to mean that you attracted or in any way deserved the abuse you've suffered from."

"I know I didn't deserve it, but I still think in some way I might have attracted it."

She shook her head. "Dawn, I think trying to understand the cause behind the events in our lives is like trying to describe the ocean by looking into a tide pool. It has personal meaning, and you can learn from it, but it's never going to give you an adequate understanding of the whole picture."

"Then how do you know what's real?"

"It's all real. Whether you actually lived those lives, or your feelings from this life were projected onto images you thought were past lives, is irrelevant. What's important, what is real, is how you feel about yourself today."

"But don't we have to understand the origin of our thoughts?"

"Whatever thoughts you came into this world with have already been reinforced by your experiences. Children who are abused feel they deserved it. They suffer from low self esteem. And most kids who are abused feel orphaned by their mothers."

"Then how do I get over it?"

"You are getting over it. You have accepted the pain of your transferences with Anne. You have looked for your disowned self in your projections. You have used your heart to feel and your intelligence to discern reality and distinguish it from illusion, and you have done all of that in the present."

"So I just stay with the program."

"I think it's working."

It was working, just not fast enough.

I left Judith's office still depressed, but with a new insight. It wasn't necessary to dig up the root to every feeling. The point of my journey was to correct the inaccurate perceptions behind the suffering so I wouldn't continue to see the world, and possibly recreate it, in the same painful way.

My isolation was becoming unbearable. No matter where I went, or who I was with, I felt alone — as if I had been shrunk and was living inside one of the glass ornaments that hung on the Christmas tree in our living room. I watched the playful activity of my family around me, but I didn't feel like a part of it.

Despite my isolation, I tried to stay in touch with my children. We had a deal that whenever they needed my attention they were to ask for their *special time*. The system kept us in sync, each of them choosing the way they wished to spend time with me. It was as if they had the power to walk into the confines of my ornament, enter my world for what they needed to give and receive, and then leave in contentment to go and play on their own.

A New Dawn Rising

The fresh oxygen my children breathed into my life kept me alive long enough to write the first thirty pages of a book: a chapter setting up the parallels between psychology and physics. After sweating over the pages until I thought I had something interesting, I took a plunge for validation and asked Philip to read it.

I handed him the chapter as I put the kids to bed. Twenty minutes later, I walked into our bedroom. He was sitting on the bed with the last page in his hand while I stood next to him anxiously waiting for a good review.

"What do you think?"

He looked up from the paper. "I love you," he said, "but this is really boring."

My head dropped so fast I pulled a muscle.

"I'm sorry," he continued, "but I think maybe you should spend some time researching the market. Find out about how people get published and what people are interested in reading."

I threw the chapter in the trash and floored myself in the nest for the rest of the evening.

In the morning, I picked myself up and went to a local bookstore. There was an older man behind the register who I assumed was the manager.

"Excuse me," I said, "do you have any information about how somebody would get a book published?"

He hummed while he thought. "No, I'm sorry, I don't, but there's a lady who works out of here a couple days a week. She's a writer and I think she just had a book picked up by a literary agent." He opened a drawer and shuffled through some papers. "Here's her card. She's a very kind woman. I'm sure she'll be helpful."

"Thank you. I'll give her a call." As I moved toward the door, a tall, well-dressed, middle-aged woman entered the store.

"Hey!" the store manager yelled. "That's her, that's the lady I was telling you about."

I looked down at her card. "Susan?"

"Yes." She reached out her hand, her eyes glowing with the clarity of a full moon.

"Hi. My name's Dawn Kohler. I'm in the process of writing a book, and I was wondering if you had any information about how somebody gets published."

She gave me a few suggestions on books I might want to read, while I grabbed a pen from my purse and wrote down the titles.

"Thank you very much. I'm starting to get my feet wet and hopefully this will give me some direction."

I looked down at her card.

```
Susan Wells
Readings
Workshops
Spiritual Counseling
```

I sensed our chance meeting was more than a coincidence, as if Susan and I were two pawns on a chessboard and the master player had just slid us into place. "Do I need to see you?" I said.

Her soft round face creased with a smile. "You'll know when you need to see me."

Of course I would. If I hadn't figured that one out by now, I never would.

I thanked her for her time and she reached out and hugged me, her embrace lifting my spirits for the rest of the day.

I ordered one of the books she suggested and pressed on, hoping to conquer my writer's block and my depression. But the words still didn't flow. Philip was right, the material was boring and even I was losing interest in it. No longer sure what I was suppose to be writing about, I stopped and asked for help. I closed my eyes that night and prayed for direction, I awoke the next morning to a vision of Susan, the woman I had met in the bookstore. I phoned her and made an appointment.

Susan's house, with its white carpet and whitewashed woods, looked more like a builder's model home than the kind of eccentric, occult domain in which I imagined a woman who did psychic readings would live. We walked into the light and airy living room. Both of us were dressed comfortably. She wore a loose cream-colored blouse with matching slacks that complimented her tall, full-body. Her face was round and soft, and her hair was short and auburn. She asked me to sit on the end of a white sofa while she pulled up a chair adjacent to me, smiling softly, as if she knew the secrets to life.

"Dawn, what I'd like to do first is just hold onto your hand for a moment while I enter into a higher state of consciousness and read your energy."

"Read my energy?"

"Yes. You might say I tap into the energy of your higher self and communicate that information back to you."

I was skeptical but intrigued.

"Just relax and don't try to think about anything you want me to pick up on. It doesn't work that way."

"Okay."

She closed her eyes and reached for my hand. A moment later her eyes opened into a stare that looked as though she was staring back into her own eyes, instead of out of them.

"Your isolation isn't over. You're in a cocoon and you need to stop trying to release yourself." Her eyes moved from side to side. "Tell the story. It will give birth to you."

"What story?"

"The story you're living. It's about our suffering and what it's for."

"I thought my book was about science and philosophy."

She smiled as her eyes cleared. "May I share with you one of the first rules I learned about writing?"

"Please."

"Don't tell people what you think, show them how you feel. That's what makes a good book, Dawn."

"But I'm still living this experience, and I'm still not sure what it's about."

"That's all right. If you're like most writers, you're not going to know what your book's about until you've finished the last chapter."

I looked at the clock. It was a half-hour session and I still had time. "Susan, if I give you the name of somebody, can you tell me about them?"

"Sure. What's the name?"

"Anne Myers."

She closed her eyes. A few moments later she went into the glazed stare and released a deep, passionate breath.

"Anne has been with you for a very long time. She's from your pod—your original family. She's here to help show you who you are."

"But she left," I said. "And I don't know if I'll ever see her again."

She shook her head. "She didn't leave. That would be impossible. She's a part of you, like a planet around your sun."

She paused for a moment. "I keep getting the image of you as a child. You're curled up in a ball, holding onto a tall, steel rod—a purpose for living while the world explodes around you."

Her eyes cleared up. "Does that image make any sense to you?"

"Yes, unfortunately, it does." I changed the subject and told her about the message I received about Anne—that when I saw Anne's soul I would see my own.

"Dawn, the image I received of you and Anne was that you are going through life back to back, but I don't get the feeling you are destined to meet again. Seeing your soul in her's might not be a literal experience."

Her words felt like a stab in my ribs. I took a deep breath. No. I would see her again. I knew I would.

Susan put her arm around my shoulders as she walked me to the door.

"Keep writing," she said. "It will help you find your way."

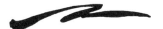

The disappointment I felt about continuing my seclusion was counterbalanced by a new sense of direction on the book. The words flowed from my fingers once I tossed research and comparisons aside and began writing the story I was living. It was the best therapy I'd had, and it gave me the confidence to write to Anne.

I spent a few days drafting a letter to bring her up to date on my process. I had waited a long time to tell her about the abuse from my dad's friends, and it felt good to finally be sharing it. Not knowing what state she was in, I kept my personal feelings light, mentioning only briefly that I wondered why I hadn't heard from her.

Karen forwarded the letter for me. Two weeks later, I received a response, opened it on the way to the nest and sat down on the daybed to read it.

Dear Dawn,

I received your letter and am amazed at all the work you've been doing. The bioenergetics work sounds great.

I am now out traveling through the states and will be for quite a while. I'm learning a lot about me and an even broader vision of life. It's very adventurous and a whole lot of fun!

I appreciate your letter. I wanted to write to also explain that I haven't contacted you because—and maybe you'll disagree with this part—I really felt I needed to stay out of your life so that you could get on with the healing. Maybe

*you feel differently—and maybe you don't anymore—but I
didn't want to interfere in any way with your therapy.*

*I hope you'll understand when I say I still think it's in
your best interest if we don't remain in contact. I hope you
always know in your heart that I care for you greatly, and
always, always wish you the very best of life.*

*This letter feels extremely inadequate for me, so I'll be
hoping this helps and not hurts you.*

Please take good, good care of yourself.

Love,
Anne

Was this good-bye, or good-bye for now? And if she had written
a letter that was adequate for her, I wondered what it would have
said. I lay back on the bed, the sun beating down on me through the
window. What about the other men? Most of my letter was about
that abuse and, she didn't even address it. I picked up the phone and
called Karen, hoping that since Anne had referred me to her, she
might have some more information about Anne.

"Karen, have you heard from Anne?"

"Why do you ask?"

"Because I received a response to my letter today, and I'm not
sure what it means."

I read Karen the note. "If it's good-bye for now," I said, "I think
she's doing the right thing, but if it's good-bye forever, I think I
deserve more than this note."

"It's your closure."

"What?"

"When Anne received your note she called me. She wasn't sure
if she should respond."

My stomach twisted into a knot. "What was she going to do, walk
away and never tell me?"

"I don't know. Because of the confidentiality between us I
couldn't advise her, but she said she realized she should have had
closure with you before she left."

"Karen, how can this note be closure? She doesn't even acknowledge the relationship."

"It sounds to me like she is trying not to hurt you."

Trying not to hurt me? I remained silent. Karen filled the gap.

"Dawn, she's moved on, and I think it's time you do the same."

"Is that what she said?"

"No, but I've known Anne for a long time and, to be honest with you, I have thought all along that you misinterpreted the relation- ship."

Misinterpreted. "Why didn't she call me? I'm the one who wrote the letter."

"I don't think she feels it would have been proper to call you. According to the ethical guidelines, if you're not her client, she should not have even responded to your letter."

"Fuck your guidelines. I'm a human being, not an object being pushed through this god-forsaken process."

"I'm sorry. I understand how you feel, but I think you need to accept things for how they are."

"How they are? Is that according to you, Anne, or some other version of this third- party communication?"

"I'm sorry, but I'm in a tough spot here."

"So am I."

I said good-bye and threw down the phone. I hated Karen at that moment, and I wasn't the least bit interested in interpreting the transference.

I read Anne's letter a hundred times. I looked at it from every angle, and the only thing that I could tell for sure was that it was consistent with what I knew of her. The letter was from the woman who cared for me greatly, remaining behind the therapist trying to play by the rules.

In my next session with Judith, I handed her Anne's note and paced across the floor as I ranted about its contents and my phone conversation with Karen. Judith sat back in her tapestry chair, hold- ing the note without unfolding it, quietly listening until I calmed down.

"Dawn, it doesn't matter what Anne's intentions behind this letter were, or how Karen interprets them. The only issue of real importance here is how you experience it." She handed me back the note. "Read it again and tell me how it makes you feel."

I read it out loud and then tossed it on the table. "It makes me feel the same way I did the day my father sent me his letter. Both of them seem content to remain at a distance , wishing me well."

"And how does that make you feel?"

"Like they don't love me enough to want to remain in my life."

"And..."

"And...like I'm not lovable enough to make them want to stay."

Judith sighed. "How much Anne and your father are capable of loving you has nothing to do with you."

"Tell that to my heart. I can reason all I want, but it still hurts like hell."

"Close your eyes."

I looked at her in protest then dropped my head into my hands.

"Bring your awareness into the pain and tell me what it says."

I took my awareness into my chest and tears began to stream from my eyes. "She didn't hear me."

"Who didn't she hear?"

"She didn't hear the six-, seven-, and eight-year-old. She didn't hear them tell her about the other men."

I opened my eyes, tears still rolling down my cheeks. "Judith, when Anne left, all she knew was that I was raped by my father. I had waited a long time to write to her about the rest of the abuse, and she didn't hear it."

Judith handed me a tissue. "Tell me more about the hurt."

"I just wanted somebody to listen to me. These men, they embarrassed me, they scared and hurt me. If I would have talked back then, I would have been killed. But now I'm safe. I can remember. I can talk, but no one's listening."

I got up again and paced the floor. "My father doesn't ever want to see me again. My mother, along with the rest of society, thinks a repressed memory is a false memory. The backlash on sexual abuse is so bad I'm embarrassed to tell anybody what I'm going through. People look at you like you've joined a therapist cult group." I grabbed another tissue, "But Anne... she was different. She had all the compassion I couldn't find in myself. She was the first person who ever made it safe enough for me to remember and who cared enough to help me through it. I believed in my heart she would always hear me."

"Just because she didn't acknowledge you doesn't mean she didn't hear."

"But she didn't share her thoughts with me. I had waited so long to tell her. I wanted to hear how she felt about it. I wanted to share her compassion. But I didn't get that, and it feels like I've been robbed." My voice started to crack. "I hate this relationship with Anne. It has so much power over me. I just want it to be over."

"Your emotions have the power over you, not Anne. Have you thought about responding to the letter?"

"What's the point? Anne's out having a good time. She doesn't want to deal with my problems."

"You need to do what's best for you, not for Anne. If it feels right to you, write her back."

I sat down and picked up the note. "Judith, what do you think of this letter?"

"I think she's ambivalent."

I looked at her for clarity.

"I think Anne has conflicting feelings for you, but that's her issue, not yours."

"Do you think she's doing this for my best interest?"

"No. I think Anne's doing this for what's in her best interest. What was in your best interest was for her to be consistent."

I stared at the floor. "I guess this means it's not all right to need her anymore."

"I can't answer that. But I don't see where it's a benefit to you."

I left Judith's office remembering what it felt like to be an eight-year-old, aimlessly walking through life, wanting somebody to do something, say something, help me through my hell, but everyone I knew was blind. I was an invisible object, filled with emotions yet walled off from my own expression or compassion.

Over the next few days, my anger and despair gave way to a burst of strength. It was time to stand up for myself. My father didn't have the conscience to listen, my mother didn't have the courage, but Anne knew better. She was capable of hearing me. And I wasn't going to let another person walk out of my life without letting them know how I felt about it.

> *Dear Anne,*
>
> *I received your letter last week. And I'm confused. I do not understand how we went from, "I'll call you when I come back" to "it's not in your best interest for us to remain in contact." I'm very hurt to think that you made such a leap in intent without at least notifying me. Certainly much has happened in both of our lives but our lack of communication has not been helpful or therapeutic. I really feel it is inappropriate for you to be making decisions based on my "best interest" without you first consulting my opinion.*
>
> *Several people have left my life this year because they did not want to deal with my feelings, and/or their own. I had hoped our relationship would be different. I*

understand the position you felt you had to take as therapist, but I do not think it should negate the fact that you and I had a very intimate bond, and went through some very real human struggles. I can respect the idea that you have moved on, but I think out of regard for the depth of our relationship, I think we both deserve more than the letter you sent.

If you want closure I will consent, but not until it's done correctly and in person. When the timing is appropriate for you, let me know. I will meet you any time, any place, to try and complete what feels to me like some very unfinished business.

Dawn

I didn't expect a response. And I didn't get one.

The weeks of summer dragged on, one day of depression leading to the next, until I stumbled across the first day of August, and the milestone of my thirty-fourth birthday. I was happy to be closing the most consciously painful year of my life, and to celebrate, I gave myself the same gift I did every year—a one-hour massage at a Ritz Carlton, a nearby resort that stood on the bluff overlooking the ocean.

I checked in at the spa desk with Jill, a slender, kind-hearted, aging hippie with straight blonde hair that fell halfway down her back, and eyes that spoke a silent wisdom. She was the senior masseuse and recognized me from previous visits.

"Hey, girl, where have you been?" she said as she handed me a towel.

"It's been a long year."

She opened the door to a dimly lit massage room and gave me a minute alone to undress. I took off my clothes and lay face down on the table. The smell of eucalyptus fragranced the air, and a flute solo playing against the sounds of the ocean came from a tape player on the floor. I let out a deep breath, then felt a warmth radiating from my body. The air in the room suddenly felt slightly humid, and for a fleeting moment, it felt as if the spirit of the Indian woman was coming from within me instead of from around me.

Jill came back in the room, pulled the sheet over my shoulders and rubbed my back in a soft spiral motion.

"Do you have any tension spots that need extra attention?"

My answer sounded muddled. My awareness had raced to the touch of her hands. My skin was still starved for the nurturing affection of a mother and I couldn't absorb her touch fast enough. I told her to focus on my shoulders while I wiped a tear from my eye.

"Are you okay?" she asked.

"I'm all right, just a little tired."

I closed my eyes. My shoulders were in knots.

"Jill, I thought I had released all this tension already. I can't believe my body is back in this condition so soon."

"Unless you have regular massages, your body is going to continue to hold blocks of tension."

"I can't justify the cost of regular massages."

"Then you should try an exercise that concentrates on releasing tension and balancing the energy in your system."

"I walk and ride my bike. Doesn't that help?"

"Sure, but it's not going to release these knots in your shoulders. Energy blocks that are created by mental tension need to be released from the inside out."

"I've been in psychotherapy for two years. Doesn't that release tension from the inside out?"

"Changing your perceptions on a thinking level is only a part of the healing process. Your perceptions do create tension, but the opposite is also true. Your tension holds in and shapes your perceptions. To change your perceptions without helping your body release the tension is only getting half the work done."

"What do you suggest?"

"Yoga or Tai Chi are good." Her fingers burrowed into my muscles.

"Do you have any instructors you recommend?"

"There are several around town—just keep your eyes open. When the student is ready, the teacher appears."

And appear he did. Three days later, I was taking my morning walk on the beach. In front of the beach club where I take the kids to swim was a Tai Chi instructor in the middle of a session. I sat and watched as he directed three women into positions that were held for several minutes. When the positions fatigued the students, I could see the shaking that started throughout their bodies. The teacher encouraged the trembling.

"When you start shaking," he said, "try to stay with it as long as possible. The muscle can no longer hold the tension and the shaking allows the body to release the blocked energy."

The postures were similar to those I'd learned in bioenergetics but concentrated more on the upper body. When the class ended, I went up and introduced myself to the instructor. Russ, an attractive man in his early thirties, with thick stubble on his face and thick, black hair combed straight back, told me he started his students with a series of exercises called the Twelve Hands of Tao Mo. Tao Mo, he explained, had been an Indian Buddhist who had spent nine years in a Shaolin temple meditating on postures to cleanse the body and enlighten the mind.

"If you're interested," he said, "you're welcome to join the class. We're here every morning at 8:30, and the exercises take about forty minutes." The timing worked with the kid's school schedules, so the next day I joined the class.

I went down early. Morning at the beach was my favorite time of the day, when the air was still and the ocean calm. I walked along the shore, deserted by people, inhabited only by birds that didn't bother to move as I passed. Russ and the other women came down from the parking lot and I walked up to meet them.

"Are you ready?" Russ said.

"I think so."

We faced the ocean as he stood in front of us and demonstrated the first position. His knees were bent, his hands straight to the side, and his fingers were spread out as far as possible. We followed him in silence. My eyes on the horizon, I felt the strong presence of the woman next to me. I knew from media coverage that her name was Denise Brown, the sister of Nicole Brown Simpson, who had been killed just two months before. Denise's mother was the second woman in the group; the third seemed to be a friend of their family. We went to the next position, our arms held out at shoulder length, our fingers spread out and pointing to the sky.

Two young boys ran up behind us. "Hey, Grandma," they yelled as they ran down to the water. One of the boys was Nicole's and O.J's son, but I didn't recognize the other. We went to the next position as the boys played in the waves. I saw the water glistening off the boy's dark skin and wondered if the ocean soothed his pain the way it used to soothe mine. As we continued the position, my legs started to shake and my hands began to tremble. Nobody else was complaining, so I endured the pain in silence.

When class was over, Denise walked up to me and introduced herself. She was polite but guarded. She asked me several questions about where I lived and what I did, and when she was confident I wasn't a reporter, she became very friendly.

"Let me introduce you to my son and nephew." She called the boys up from the water and I tensed as Nicole's five-year-old son approached us. I had been told several times that I resembled his mother, and I was concerned that my presence might confuse him.

Before I could excuse myself, he saw me standing next to his aunt and grandmother on the same beach where he'd often seen his mother. My long, blonde hair was enough to give him hope and, from a hundred feet away we locked eyes — I seeing something strangely familiar in him, him desperate to see his mother in me. I wanted to say, "I'm sorry I'm not her," but his mind was already caught in the confusion. In his eyes, I could see his hope turned to disappointment, despair, then a rage that brought tears to us both. I wasn't who he needed me to be. He turned and ran back into the water.

The other women were talking and the event went unnoticed, but I'll never forget his face or the torment that glazed his dark-brown eyes.

My next session with Judith was more depressing than usual as I told her about my encounter with Nicole's son.

"Dawn, you said you saw his pain. What did you see?"

His dark face was etched in my mind. "He's holding his breath. Deep in his heart, he's holding his breath, waiting for his mother to return."

She stared at me. "Who are you holding your breath for?"

My stomach dropped to the floor. "I hate it when you do that," I said.

"That doesn't answer the question."

I looked down. "When you're a child, you hope. You hope that someday the people who have left your life will reappear, love you the way you need to be loved, and everything that happened will fade like a bad dream."

"And what happens if you stop holding your breath? If you let go of the hope?"

"I'll die. If I give up the hope, I can't survive."

She leaned forward. "You can't survive? Or the five-year-old child inside of you can't survive?"

"Both."

"Are you still waiting for Anne to return?"

"I know it doesn't make sense, but waiting for Anne to return goes much deeper than Anne. I'm waiting for a part of me to return, and I have to believe, I have to hope that someday that's going to happen."

"And what if it doesn't? What if, just like that little boy, you have to realize that she's never coming back?"

"Then I don't know what will happen to me."

"Dawn, you took Anne for your mother. And there is no hope that she will ever be your mother. You need to realize that."

"I know she wasn't my mother, but the need for her is still so strong."

Judith sat back and put a lozenge in her month. "Close your eyes," she said.

"Why?"

"Just do it."

I was tired of doing guiding imagery, tired of feeling like a five-year-old. I closed my eyes and took a deep breath.

"I want you to go to your garden and ask a child to appear. When you have someone, let me know."

In my mind, I entered the wood garden gate and found two children sitting on the white bench. The first child was me as a five-year-old, still wearing my black turtleneck and blue jeans, sitting with one knee up under her arm. The second was me at the age of eight. My permanent teeth had come in, and my bangs were cut an inch above my eyebrows. I gave Judith the description.

"The five-year-old looks lonely and the eight-year-old is scared, distant."

"Ask them why they feel that way."

"The five-year-old needs Anne—she wants somebody safe to love. And the eight-year-old is afraid. Afraid she's going to die. She still thinks the men are going to kill her."

Judith cleared her throat. "Dawn, I want you to bring yourself into the image as an adult and take the two children in your lap. When they're comfortable I want you to show them a photo album. Show them pictures of Philip, Samantha, Michael, and Erica. Show the five-year-old all the people in her life that she can safely give her love to. And then show the eight-year-old pictures to let her know she grew up. She's safe now; the men didn't kill her."

In my mind, I took the two children in my lap and opened the photo album. The first picture that appeared was the Polaroid of the dead girl lying naked on the floor, her throat slit from ear to ear. My heart started to race and my hands sweated profusely.

"Judith, it's the picture they showed me to keep me quiet. These men are going to kill me. I'm not safe! I'm not safe anywhere!"

"You're all right and you're safe. Tell me what you're experiencing."

I started to cry. "The child in this picture was killed. She was murdered. " I felt the terror she felt before her death, the terror I numbed out when they threatened my life by holding the picture in front of me.

I opened my eyes and jumped to my feet. "They're going to kill me. I knew too much. I played along so they wouldn't hurt me, but I still knew too much." I paced the floor. "I never knew when they were going to change their minds. When they had had enough of me. I never knew when they were going to kill me."

"Dawn, they didn't kill you. You grew up. It's over."

"It's never over! It's inside of me every day!" I grabbed a pillow and held it to my chest. "Why did my dad do this to me? Damn him! Why?"

Judith was silent.

"I've had enough!" I said. "I'm not going to be safe until he's dead. Until I kill him."

"How would you kill him?"

"With a shotgun. I'd walk into his office, point it to his head and send him to hell the hard way."

Judith pulled out a box of crayons and a large pad of paper.

"Come sit on the floor. Pick out a crayon and draw me a picture of your father."

I pulled out a thick red crayon and drew my dad.

"Now draw the gun," she said. I drew of picture of myself pointing a shotgun in his face. "You've got the gun to his head. What do you want him to say to you?"

"I'm sorry. I want him to acknowledge my pain and say he's sorry."

"Write it."

I drew a line from his month. In big, red letters I wrote:

I'M SORRY, DAWN. I'M SORRY!

"What do you want to do next?"

"Kill him."

"Then kill him." I took my red crayon and crossed him out of my life like the death of a bad dream. When his picture was nothing more than a blotch of red wax, I doubled over and sobbed.

"He's dead, Dawn. He can't hurt you anymore."

I gasped for air. "I love you, Dad. I love you."

Chapter 10

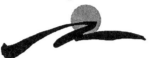

The cells in my body felt as if they were slowly melting, being drained like a glass jar full of dirty grease and scrubbed clean so I could receive something new. I continued to write the story as it unfolded, hoping that it would lead to some clarity. In the meantime, I followed the path—a road paved by my daily events and encounters that compelled me to keep moving.

The last week in August, Phil and I received an invitation to a wedding being held in late September. Jon, the last of our high school friends to get married, was having the ceremony and reception in McCall, a resort town in Idaho. I booked our reservations and confirmed our travel plans.

The long days of summer were coming to an end. Phil had closed down the ICON building, and the clients and staff were up and running with the new parent company. The final check for the acquisition was to clear the bank in a week, and Phil was planning to quit his job as soon as the funds hit our account.

The summer was so hectic we barely spoke. The kids kept us in communication, but, apart from providing for their needs, we were as far apart as we had ever been. I spent my evenings writing at my computer; Phil spent his in the garage cutting out the inside of an old cargo van and building what looked like a bed across the back. I walked into the garage one night when he was about halfway through the project.

"What are you building?" I asked.

"A dog van." He revved up his power drill.

"What for?"

"When I quit next week, Maxx and I are going on a fishing trip."

"For how long?"

He turned off the drill. "Indefinitely."

"Excuse me?"

"Indefinitely." He leaned up against the van. "Dawn, for the past two years I've taken care of your company, your kids, and you. Now it's time I take care of myself."

"Where are you going?"

"I'm heading north. You can meet me in Idaho for Jon's wedding, then I'll probably go into the Sierras for a while."

"When are you coming home?"

"I don't know. But every time you ask me, the trip is going to get longer."

I leaned up against his workbench. An indefinite fishing trip sounded a little too close to an indefinite sabbatical for me, but I knew for the kids' sake, he wouldn't be gone too long.

The next morning, I went down to my Tai Chi class. Russ led the Twelve Hands exercise in silence. Denise stood next to me. Occasionally, I'd see tears running down her face. Occasionally, she'd see tears running down mine.

The postures flushed up more emotions. I felt tired of the suffering. It had been a year since Anne left, and my yearnings to see her were growing; our relationship still felt terribly incomplete. Russ moved to the next position, our arms extended above our heads pushing flat palms to the sky as if we were holding up a ceiling. I stared out at the ocean. Where was this path taking me, and how much longer could I stand to be on it?

I met Judith that afternoon. Her office looked colorless. I took my seat feeling as if I was sitting down to a bland meal, a meal I had eaten too many times.

"Judith, does this pain ever end?"

"Pain is part of the human condition."

"Does that mean it's not going to end?"

"No, I think we have the capacity to transcend our suffering, but pain is a psychological response; as long as you are a human being you will be vulnerable to pain."

"But is there a cure?"

"I don't promise cures, but you will feel better."

My shoulders drooped, "God, I miss Anne."

"Why's that?"

"She told me I'd be healed and I believed her."

She nodded. "That reminds me. Did you get a response to your letter?"

"No...I didn't."

"Maybe she didn't receive it," Judith said.

"She got it. Whenever she receives something from me, my chest warms and I know."

"If you know she received your letter, how does it make you feel that she didn't respond to it?"

"I didn't expect her to."

"Yes, but how does her not responding to your letter make you feel?"

I let the question sink in. "Ashamed."

"What are you ashamed of?"

"Me. I don't know if I have told you this, but the last day I saw Anne, she held me in her arms for most of the session. I had never let anybody close enough to me to hold me like that, and afterwards it embarrassed me."

"How did it embarrass you?"

"When my walls were down, when Anne had the chance to see me for who I am, I think she saw something very ugly. Something so disgraceful that she didn't want to see me again."

Judith winced. "You're describing shame. The feeling that at the core of our being we are ugly and undesirable."

"Ugly, worthless, humiliated. Anne not staying in contact with me makes me feel the way I did when my dad molested me. He didn't want to talk to me either. I was so ugly it made him go away, and it feels like whatever my dad saw in me, Anne saw, too."

"That sounds very painful."

"It makes me so disgusted with myself, I want to leave my own body."

Judith looked angry, and I was getting the impression she was starting not to like Anne. "Do you understand that your vulnerability with Anne had nothing to do with her leaving? The shame you feel is the legacy your father handed down to you. It's a feeling, but who you are is not your feelings of shame. You are not ugly or unlovable."

"Yes, I do understand that, but it's like everything else I have experienced. Knowing a truth is only the first stage of actually realizing it."

Judith paused. "Do you know where you feel the shame in your body?"

"It starts in my chest and it goes to the seat of my pelvis."

"Do you want to do a guided imagery?"

The depths of my shame were the depths of my hell and I wasn't all that eager to go there. "No. I'm too tired."

"Okay, you go at your own pace."

"Judith, do you think I'm ever going to hear from Anne again?"

"I don't know, but if you don't, you shouldn't take it personally. How other people handle their relationships has nothing to do with you as a person. It's how they are in the world, and it's not about you.

"That's a hard one for me."

"That's a hard one for everyone."

The first Monday in September we received a cashier's check for the sale of ICON. Philip cashed the check at lunch and quit his job that afternoon. He came home with a six-pack of beer and a can of lighter fluid. "Come on kids, we're building a fire."

We all followed him out to the back yard where he handed the garden hose to Michael, threw his shirt, tie and brown leather shoes in the center of the lawn and drenched the pile with lighter fluid. When he tossed in a burning cigar, a five-foot flame rose from the fire. Our yard smelled like a Tijuana trash fire as Phil cracked opened his beer and started to sing, "You can take this job and shove it, I ain't working here no more." After he finished his beer, Philip and Michael doused the fire.

"Come on kids, we're going to Toys-R-Us!"

We all jumped in the car and headed to the strip mall. With two carts we ran through the store, the kids filling the baskets with balls, water guns, dolls, and action figures.

"Next stop," Phil yelled, "Sport Mart!"

We filled another basket at Sport Mart with lures, rods, and hiking gear. Then we came home and helped Phil pack the dog van.The next morning Phil and Maxx were ready to leave. Maxx licked my face as I said good-bye to him; we walked together every day and I was going to miss that dog as much as I'd miss Phil.

Phil loaded Maxx in the van and gave me a kiss. I wanted to ask when he was coming home, but didn't. I just told him I loved him and let him go.

The kids seemed secure with the fate of our family. The only sign of rebellion was an expression of Michael's. I came home one day to find a large letter "M" written in blue crayon across the white garage door. I walked in the back door and found Michael in the family room watching T.V. On the floor next to him was the same blue crayon that he'd used to tag the door. "Michael, did you draw the "M" on the garage door?"

He looked me right in the eye. "No, Mom, it wasn't me."

"Do you think Erica or Samantha would have written a large "M" on the garage door?"

"Maybe they were trying to write Mom," he said as he nonchalantly turned his head back toward the TV. I turned off the television and took him by the hand to go scrub the door. "If you're going to tag, son, never use your own initials."

I avoided the subject of shame for my next two sessions. Judith let me dance around it while I adjusted to Phil's absence. When I ran out of current issues, she slyly brought it up.

"Do you know where you need to go next?"

I smiled. "Yes, we both know where I need to go next."

"Do you still feel the shame in your chest?"

"Yes, and it feels as if this love I feel for Anne, this growing torch in my body, seems to be dredging the shame up."

She raised an eyebrow and grinned. "Close your eyes."

"You like this don't you?"

"Not as much as you'd think."

I took a deep breath and leaned my head back against the chair.

"Bring your awareness into the area you describe in your chest and when you have settled there for a moment, tell me what you see and feel."

After a few moments of silence, I felt a pull drawing me into a cave that opened at the center of my chest. The entrance was large and dark; fresh water dripped from the sides of the walls. A chill ran through my body and a seductive thirst pulled me more deeply into the cave. Elisa, the seated Indian woman appeared, her brown face serene in the half-light of the cave.

Stop resisting, stop resisting.

I let go of my desire to stay at the entrance of the cave and felt the sensation of being sucked into its vortex. Pulled into its core, my body suddenly felt horizontal, as if I was lying flat on my back, buried alive in a six-foot grave.

"Judith, I'm in a grave."I tried to dig my way out.

"Dawn, ask Elisa what this image is all about."

Let go, let go of your life.

I repeated the message to Judith and told her I was fighting it.

"Fight as long as you need to," she said. My father and Anne appeared on the top of my grave. I clinched my jaw, tightened my fists and fought to pull them in with me. Reaching to the surface, I grabbed my father's shirt, but when I touched him, his image disappeared. I reached behind him toward Anne, but the minute I touched her, she too was gone. I lay back in my grave, fighting until I was exhausted, and finally I gave up.

I felt myself return to the sensation of being horizontal.In my mind, I looked around and saw that I was now on a small platform going down into a well. The image of the well's deep shaft felt like it opened in my chest and ran down my torso to the floor of my body. It was dark and stuffy, and the platform I was on suspended me, inside the well in my body, at a level just above my sternum. I described the image to Judith.

"Dawn, ask Elisa to tell you more about where you are."

"The grave shows me that I need to let go of my life. The well represents a new transition."

"Ask Elisa what you need to do next."

Stay in the well. Be aware.

I repeated the message to Judith, then shot opened my eyes. "Do you think I'm really going to die?"

"Someday."

"I don't like this, Judith. It scares me."

"What scares you about it?"

"Judith, I'm on a platform that's going down into a well in my body, and Elisa just told me to let go of my life. I don't want to let go of my life."

"I think it's just a metaphor. Throughout mythology you can see the process of transformation illustrated by the images of towers, caves, castles, and wells. It's these dark, scary places that the heroes enter to retrieve lost parts of themselves."

"Yes, if the dark, scary places doesn't kill them."

She smiled. "Just remember what Elisa said — stay in the well and pay attention."

"Are you sure I'm not going to die?"

"I don't know. I left my crystal ball at home."

I winced in frustration. "You're not very comforting."

"You're in a well. I don't think you're supposed to be comfortable."

I sat back in my chair, hoping she'd say something compassionate, hoping she'd say something Anne would say. She didn't, so I stood up to leave.

"Dawn, there's one more thing I want you to do this week."

"What's that?"

"Write Anne's eulogy."

"What?"

"It's time, Dawn. If you ever see Anne again, you and she will be different people. The relationship you had is over, and it's time you had closure."

"When I see her again, I'll have closure."

"Write the eulogy."

"I'll think about it."

That weekend was Jon's wedding, and some friends and I boarded a plane for Idaho to meet up with Philip as planned. I was over my fear of flying, the white-knuckled flights I use to take in college, but under the circumstances I was still anxious — being told to let go of your life isn't the kind of message you want to receive just before boarding a plane.

We landed safely in Boise and rented a car to drive to McCall. Two hours later we arrived at the lakefront resort, a renovated hunting lodge wrapped around the end of a cove, nestled between the tall pines that lined the shore of the lake. I checked into our hotel and walked down to the dock. The air was like a splash of cool water, the sky so blue it looked animated.

I spotted Phil sitting on the dock, a fishing pole in one hand, a beer in the other, and Maxx lying next to him. I picked up a rock and lobbed it by his line. Phil looked for the fish. Maxx raced toward me.

"Hi, boy," I said as he jumped all over me.

Philip reeled in his line and got up to hug me. "Get out of there, Maxx, she's my chick."

I wrapped my arms around him. His body felt hard, his eyes lonely.

"Did you miss me?" I said.

"I think about you all the time," he replied.

We put Maxx in the van and walked into our room. He shut the door behind us and pulled me into his arms, his kiss arousing my need to be loved. But his touch was rough, more aggressive than loving. It was too much, too fast, and before I knew it I was naked on my back, tears rolling into my ears.

Phil slid off me. "I'm sorry," he said, "but it's just been so long."

"I know." He put his arm around my waist. I closed my eyes, I felt myself sliding deeper into the well. The loneliness was excruciating.

"Everybody's meeting at a bar up the street," he said. "Do you want to go?"

"Sure." We showered and walked into town, and by the time we entered the bar it looked like a high school reunion. The first person to greet me was Mary, the bridegroom's mother. Mary was a retired professor of medical genetics, a handsome gray-haired woman with the sturdy body of a mountain hiker and the soft lines of a woman aging gracefully. Her tan face and her clear, blue-water eyes both lit up as she recognized me.

"Motherhood must be agreeing with you," she said. "You look very different." She stared at me for several moments while other friends came up to greet me. When the conversation hit a lull, she pulled me aside.

"Tell me what's happening to you." Was she asking about the incest?

"What do you mean?" I asked.

"You look different. Your eyes have more clarity." I sensed from the clarity in her own eyes that she was referring to my spiritual path. I told her I had been feeling some changes in my body, deep vibrations at night. Her eyes continued to sparkle so I went a little further and told her about the messages I had been receiving from images that spontaneously arose in my mind. And I mentioned the various coincidences, like meeting Susan in the bookstore that continued to lead me. She smiled widely.

"You're having a spiritual awakening," she said. "I retired fifteen years ago, and I've been studying the process of transformation ever since. It's the most exciting thing I've ever done."

"It's exciting, all right."

"Oh, Dawn, this is the most wonderful time to be alive. The spiritual elements being discovered in physics, astronomy, psychology, and neurobiology are fascinating." She elaborated on a theory in neurobiology. Seeing it was over my head, she slowed down and went back to common ground.

"Did your spiritual awakening begin spontaneously, or did something trigger it?" she asked.

"I don't know. I just woke up one morning with a ball of energy in the center of my chest, and then all hell broke loose."

Philip came up and joined the conversation while Mary grabbed a pen from her purse and took down my address.

"I would love to talk to you more about this. I have built a wonderful home in San Luis Obispo. It would be great fun if you could come up and visit."

I thanked her for the invitation and went in to the party, apprehensive about seeing old friends. The word had gotten around about the abuse, and I wasn't sure if my suffering would be acknowledged or if my encounters would be awkward.

Phil and I stood at the bar as friends approached. To my delight, it was never awkward; whether in a warm, deep embrace or in words of condolence, everybody who knew acknowledged my pain, repeating sentiments I had heard from others. "We always knew you were running from something. We just didn't know what."

The wedding was held in an old, refurbished barn, the walls paneled with pinewood, the back doors converted to a pane-glass window that looked over a wheat field and into a meadow. In front of the window was the altar, and the ceremony began with Jennifer's maid of honor reciting an excerpt from *The Prophet* by Kalil Khabran:

GIVE YOUR HEARTS, BUT NOT INTO EACH OTHER'S KEEPING.
FOR ONLY THE HAND OF LIFE CAN CONTAIN YOUR HEARTS.

AND STAND TOGETHER YET NOT TOO NEAR TOGETHER:
FOR THE PILLARS OF THE TEMPLE STAND APART,
AND THE OAK TREE AND THE CYPRESS, GROW NOT IN EACH
OTHER'S SHADOW.

I smiled at Phil as we stood against a beam. He raised an eyebrow and nodded.

The vows were exchanged, the bride and groom kissed, and for the next ten hours we sang, danced and laughed at Maxx lapping up the spilled beer on the barn floor, getting as drunk as Phil. At midnight, I lifted the car keys from Phil's pocket. He was on his twenty-something beer, and we were about to begin our usual routine.

"Hey, I can drive," he said in a slurred voice.

"I'm sure you can, but I need the practice."

I rounded up Maxx and put him in the van while Phil staggered into the front seat and hung his head out the window. The map was on the floor, and I picked it up as we left the parking lot; five miles later we were lost. I pulled over and turned on the light. It was forty degrees out and I was freezing, but Phil had passed out against the door, and I didn't dare close the window. The only thing worse than throwing up myself was watching somebody else do it.

Maxx came up from the back and licked my face.

"God, Maxx, even you smell like beer." I pushed him away. "Go sit down, boy."

I picked up the directions again. Turn left at the tree stump, right at the end of the Murphy's green barn. It was pitch black out. How was I supposed to find a tree stump? I rolled up the map and hit Phil over the head.

"Will you get up?" I yelled.

He didn't move.

For the next hour I was lost, driving down dark rural streets in Idaho, my lips turning blue from the cold as Phil snored. I yelled at him some more.

"Why do you do this?" I screamed. "Why do I do this?"

I finally found a main street and followed a truck into town and pulled into the hotel parking lot exhausted. I tried to move Phil. He didn't budge, so I threw a blanket over him and locked the car, figuring he had had too much alcohol in him to freeze to death.

On Sunday I rolled over and crawled out of bed. Sometime during the night, Phil had made it to our room.

"I'm getting too old for this," I said.

"What? Just because you had to drive me home."

I wasn't in the mood for a fight. We went out to breakfast with the couple I'd flown up with. After we ate, Phil walked us out to the cars. Neither one of us was sure where our marriage was headed, if the path I was on was going to pull us apart, or somehow take us to a new place so we could finally be together. He opened my car door and said goodbye, looking at me as if the person he married wasn't coming back. I closed the door not feeling much of anything. He drove into the Sierras and I headed for the airport and home to my well.

On the flight home, I closed my eyes and checked in with my inner world. The platform I was on had sunken to a lower level and

Elisa, the seated Indian woman draped in an orange shawl, was at the top of the shaft.

Pay attention. Stay aware.

I felt a subtle dread in the pit of my stomach. I had descended further from the light. The well was getting darker and the damp, cold chill that ran through my body gave me the sense that I was going through a spiritual hazing and the obstacles were about to get tougher. I slept poorly that night and woke up to the phone ringing. The housekeeper was calling in sick, and my mother was scheduled for a visit.

Mom came up once a month to see her grandchildren, and I normally left an hour before she arrived and returned only after I knew she was gone. But with the housekeeper out for the day, there was no one else to stay with the children, so for the first time in eight months, I was going to have to see my mother.

I struggled through the morning picking up clothes and putting away dishes, fueling my anger with every breath. How could I stay civil? She'd betrayed me as child, as an adult, as a human being, and now with the full knowledge of the abuse in my childhood, I would have to face her once again.

At eleven o'clock, the bell rang and Erica ran to open the door. My mother walked in wearing a bright yellow pantsuit, carrying a bouquet of fresh cut flowers.

"It's so good to see you, baby," she said as she threw her arms around me.

I felt like I'd just landed in the twilight zone.

"You look good honey. Are you feeling better?" she said.

"I'm working on it."

"I think about you all the time, and I hope you know I love you."

Who was this lady? "The kids are upstairs," I said. "I have some errands to run."

"Don't rush. Take all the time you need." She unloaded a bag of presents while I walked slowly out of the house.

Didn't I hate her? Maybe not. Maybe I'd forgotten about the good things, the parts of her I loved. She was warm, attractive, and generous. She loved and nurtured my children. And she genuinely seemed to care about me. Was this the same mother I'd spoken to eight months ago on the phone? The woman who would rather believe an Oprah show than me?

I couldn't remember what I was shopping for, so I drove to a friend's house, borrowed a room, and took a nap. Three hours later I woke up just as confused, just as tired.

I drove home to relieve my mom of the children. When I pulled up in the driveway, they were all out front playing ball, the kids' faces smeared with homemade chocolate chip cookies. Mom came up and kissed me good-bye.

"Honey, if you ever need me, you know I'll be there."

I stared at her as she got in her car. *What! I did need you. You weren't there. You're cold, ignorant, and defensive. Why are you acting like you're not?*

I went in the house and put a video in for the kids, then retreated into my room and called Judith.

She returned my call within the hour. "Dawn, I'm sure your mother is a compassionate woman who loves you and your children deeply. And she can also be cold, narrow-minded and defensive. It's not a black-and-white world. Both sides of your mother exist."

"Then why am I so confused?"

"Because as a child you tried to make sense of the world by seeing it in terms of black and white, all or nothing, good and evil. But both good and bad traits exist in people. It's the same principle we discussed in regard to your father."

"But her words are so different from her actions, they seem to be coming from two different value systems."

"Because they do. People have different values for different situations. Your mother's compassion in one situation is as real as her defensiveness and denial in another. Both traits exist, and you need to keep telling yourself that."

Judith repeated herself several times but her answer didn't satisfy me. I hung up the phone in frustration and lay back in my bed. Why had she changed? Why was she at times a defensive, ill-informed, neglectful mother and other times an understanding and compassionate one? I remembered the day in the bathroom when I'd screamed for her help, the times my frustration with her drinking had fallen on deaf ears, and the abuse memories I had tried to explain to her. If my mother really loved me, why had she continually turned away? Why had she denied my pain?

For the next week I wallowed in self-pity — the isolated pit of neglect where I went when my wounds were not acknowledged or understood. My body tensed all day with anger. At night I'd curl up in my sheets and cry myself to sleep. By the end of the week I was exhausted, but as I laid myself down to bed one night, I felt the pain subside and a revelation emerged. My mother wasn't denying my pain — she was denying her own. The way she knew how to love me was real, but limited to the way she chose to see the world, and her limitations, needing to protect her relationship with my father, instead of protecting me, had nothing to do with me as a person. My muscles and breath released and my body fell into a deep sleep.

In the morning, I checked into the well in my inner world. I had descended to a level just above my belly button. At the top of the shaft was Madame, the majestic wise woman with the long, white cape and high-pointed collar. I acknowledged her presence and went about my day.

I took the kids to school and went to the beach for my exercise class. The Browns had quit to attend the trial, and a few friends from my neighborhood had taken their places. When class was over my neighbors and I walked down the beach. Aurora, a Costa Rican woman in her mid-forties, brought up the Simpson trial. Despite the evidence, she would not entertain the possibility that O.J. Simpson could have committed the murders of Ron Goldman and Nicole Brown Simpson.

"It's a mistake," she said. "The whole thing is just a mistake."

"That his DNA matched with blood at the murder scene was a mistake?" I said.

"That doesn't prove anything."

The rage welled up in my face as we started to argue over the evidence. Socks, shoes, blazers, motive—none of it meant a thing to her. I dropped into emotions I rarely displayed outside of therapy, but the harder I fought for her to acknowledge the possibility of Mr. Simpson's guilt, the harder she fought to deny it. Toxic with rage, I abruptly ended the argument, walked away, and came home trying to calm myself down.

Who was I fighting? Aurora, my mother, or myself?

On my bed, I closed my eyes and took a few deep breaths. The well appeared and I looked up from the platform to see Madame, standing stoic in her long, white cape. What was that about? I asked.

If you can't teach, walk away.

My anger turned to humility. There was a big difference between educating people and threatening their defenses, and I was obviously doing the latter. I descended to a lower, narrower level of the well.

The week had aroused in me a passionate hostility toward my mother—and now Aurora. The emotions were uncomfortable, and I wanted to resolve them, so I went to my desk and wrote down what enraged me.

*They are narrow-minded.*Remembering the projection rule, I re-wrote it in the first person. *I am narrow-minded.* No way! I was well-read and willing to learn. I was willing to challenge my beliefs with emerging information. I stayed open to all possibilities. So why was I fighting this so hard?

After exhausting my first reaction, I took a more honest look. Until a few years ago, I hadn't read much of anything other than the *Wall Street Journal*. I was a Reaganomics Republican who thought all human suffering was caused by lazy, bleeding-heart liberals who needed to quit whining and get a job. And I was notorious for gauging people by their behavior, believing the only true measure of a person's character was hard work and productivity. From the way I saw my family to the way I saw the world, my life had been based on narrow-minded perspectives that denied the pain of others, all in an effort to deny my own pain.

To let go of the past, I had to come to terms with it, accept myself for what I had been, and appreciate the benefits of my denial. My narrow-minded defenses had kept me from feeling the depths of my abuse, and until I was in a safe place, with safe people, it would have killed me to unleash it.

Philip called that week. He missed the kids and the kids missed him, but we both knew it wasn't time for us to be together again.

When we got off the phone, I put the kids to bed and went to my room to lie down and check in to the inner world of the well. A few moments after closing my eyes, the image of me standing on an old wood scaffolding in a cold, dark, well appeared. I felt cramped and damp. I had reached the narrow bottom, only inches above the water. The light from the top looked like a distant glow. To drop much further would mean my death, and I was taking the idea literally again. In a panic, I called Judith for some comfort, and maybe for an extra appointment. She called back. She didn't think it was necessary to see me, nor did she offer me any words of comfort. I hung up frustrated. Her response, by intention, was as cold as the well.

My fear of death escalated through the week, and by Sunday morning, I was too nervous to eat.

"Mom, there's a rat on the patio," Michael said as he stared out the kitchen window.

I looked out the French doors to the back yard. Three feet from the pane was a huge, gray tree rat sitting on the brick patio, staring at the door. The kids and I tapped on the glass, rattled the window and yelled as loud as we could, but the rat just sat there, blinking its eyes, looking as if it was struggling for breath.

Why was this happening? We had lived in that house for five years, and never before had an animal come up to our back door to die. Was this an omen, or was pest control in the neighborhood? We checked on the tree rat throughout the day. At sunset, we found the rat's fury, gray, body had fallen over dead. The rattle of death was now at my door, and I was running out of places to hide.

The next day I awoke in a sweat, jumped out of bed and distracted myself with errands. In the afternoon I returned home with Erica, the animated look in her big, blue eyes, and her red pigtails and freckle-covered face, seemed to calm me down. I put her down in the playroom for some quiet time and went into my room to read.

Twenty minutes later, my door opened and Erica peered around the corner. "I have a present for you," she said. In her hand was a gift she had wrapped with typing paper and a roll of scotch tape. "Open it."

It took me several minutes to tear through the tape and the paper and uncover the backside of an old paperback book. I turned it over and read the titled: *Denial of Death* by Ernest Becker. A chill ran up my spine.

"Erica, where did you find this?"

"Under the couch."

I covered up my panic, gave her a kiss, and sent her back to the playroom. A neighbor had given me the book several years before. It must have gotten lost in the playroom. But it didn't mean anything, finding a book on death. It was just a coincidence. Just a very strange, eerie coincidence.

I jumped out of bed and ran some more errands. Erica and I picked Michael up from his friend's house, met Samantha at school and then went to the video store. I browsed through the racks, looking for something light, something that would bring me back to my senses. The kids picked out a cartoon and I picked up the romantic comedy *Sleepless in Seattle*. I hadn't seen the movie, but I was hopeful that Tom Hanks and Meg Ryan could pull me out of my despair.

We went home to do homework, eat dinner, take baths, and make popcorn.

By movie time, the kids were clean and nestled by my side, all of us wrapped in a blanket on the big green couch. I took a deep breath. I was safe, needed, and probably not going to die. Samantha got up to start the movie, and the opening scene appeared Tom Hanks playing a man standing at the grave of his dead wife. I thought I was going to lose my mind — the image of the grave filled my body with terror.

"Mom, what's he doing? Where's he at?"

My heart was pounding through my ears.

"Mom, did that little boy's mom die?" Samantha said.

"Can that really happen?" Michael asked.

The rat, the book, and now *Sleepless in Seattle.* If there was anything I'd learned from my mother, it was that omens came in threes. I did my best to answer their questions and caught my tears in a handful of toilet paper through the rest of the movie.

When the video was over, I tucked the girls into bed and walked into Michael's room. I was trying not to cry as I kissed him good-night, but the thought of dying and leaving him motherless was more than I could bear. Tears streamed down my face.

"What's wrong, Mom?"

"I'm just tired. That's all, honey, I'm just very tired."

He handed me his red Power Ranger doll. "Don't worry, Mom, he'll protect you."

I reached down and picked my son up in my arms. "I love you so much, Michael." We held each other, then I gently put him down on his pillow and kissed him goodnight.

It was my darkest hour. Too tired to sleep, too scared to move, I walked into the nest, curled up in a ball, and let the anguish of my pending death overcome me.

If you're going to take me, God, take me now. I can't stand this any longer.

I closed my eyes and waited to die. And in that moment, in the abyss of my mind, in a terror that was inhuman, I found myself. I found myself in the same place I had been my entire life. Curled up in a ball, in the pit of my stomach, in a well full of shame, afraid I was going to die. I let go of myself and started to cry.

My life had been spared. The terror in my body ebbed and peace flowed over me as the image of the well appeared, and a gold staircase arose from the walls.

Release yourself.

With elation, I climbed to the top.

Chapter 11

Judith embraced me as I entered her office, holding me tightly, giving me the comfort she somehow knew she couldn't give me while I worked through the issues that had been represented in the well.

"I feel empty," I said as I plopped down in my chair. "And my body aches, as if I am chemically addicted to the well and I'm craving to crawl back into it.

"You've been in that well most of your life. It's natural that you would feel pulled to go back to the only place you've ever known."

"But I feel toxic, like the well's heavy, polluted smell is clinging to me."

She nodded. "If you took an object from a well where it had been for thirty years, the object would still have the smell and the energy of the well."

"Then how do I cleanse myself?"

"Close your eyes."

I looked at her. "You don't believe in much foreplay, do you?"

"I thought we did have foreplay."

"I guess it's all in the perception."

She laughed, and told me to take a few deep breaths and go to the image of the well. On my second breath, I saw the image of me sitting on a patch of green grass next to a deep hole in the ground, my body yearning to jump in.

"I want you to ask either Elisa or Madame to come in and give you some guidance." Madame appeared by my side. Her small, handsome face looked serious and dignified.

Do not return to the well.

An iron grate slammed down over the hole. Through a telepathic thought, Madame told me to follow her. She led me down a path that began several yards from the well. The heavy vegetation of a tropical forest began to appear as we walked through a warm, light-gray mist held in by the tall fan palms that filtered in long streams of soft, white light. After several minutes, we came to a natural pool of water. The pool was fed by a clear waterfall that cascaded like melted glass over a six-foot ledge. At the other end of the pond were small rock streams that drained the pool into a creek below it. I bent down and touched the water; it felt like tepid, liquid silk and left a light, gold sheen on my hands. Madame walked me back to the well.

"Dawn, what's happening?" Judith asked.

"Madame showed me a pool to cleanse in. I'm to sit by the well and take baths in the pool."

"How often are you supposed to do this?"

"Whenever I feel dirty."

"Good. Bring in whatever you'll need to be comfortable." I imagined myself naked in a big, white, cotton robe and then brought in the image of my blue, high-back beach chair to sit in while I stayed by the well.

"Is there anything else you need to know, or take with you, before we wrap up?"

Madame stood by my side. *You will shine again.*

I brought my consciousness back into the office.

"What do you think?" I said.

"I think you're in the process of mourning the process. There is a very real loss involved when we transform out of old familiar ways of being in the world."

"Judith, I thought when I found myself, I would feel whole."

"You're still in the process."

"I'm sick of the process."

Judith smiled. "Then go bathe in your pool." She got up and hugged me. "Hang in there—you're doing good work."

I went home for lunch but couldn't eat, my body felt as though I had inhaled the fumes from an oil refinery. I took a couple aspirin, went up to the nest and lay down on the bed until the well appeared.

When it did, I walked back to the pool and took off my robe. The air felt balmy and the tall vegetation that shaded the pool gave me a sense of protection. I stepped into the water and waded under the falls, the warm liquid caressing my hair, washing my face and massaging my neck and shoulders. It felt as though a refreshing peace was pouring through my body, as though...

"Mom, we're home!" Michael screamed through the doorway. The image disappeared.

"Can I have something to eat?" Erica yelled right behind him.

The mother from the car pool came up to the door. "Are you home?"

"Yes, I'm here. Thanks for picking them up," I said.

I jumped up to go downstairs, feeling lighter, cleaner, *hungry*.

I gave the kids a bath that night. The phone rang while I was rinsing their hair, so I put Samantha in charge and ran to answer it.

"Hi," Phil said. "Can I come home yet?"

I sat down on the bed.

"Where are you?"

"I'm on the freeway, about an hour north."

There was a long silence. "I want you to come home," I said, "but...I'm still not ready to be with you."

Another long silence. "That's okay. How about if I come home and take care of the kids and you can take Maxx and go someplace?"

"That sounds good." I hung up the phone and went back to the kids. A week away would be nice. It would give me time alone to bathe in my pool, to cleanse the layers of pollutants I still felt in my body.

That week I received a package from Mary, Jon's mother with whom I reunited at his wedding in Idaho. The box included a book on spiritual healing and an open invitation to visit her in San Luis Obispo. I knew from our encounter in Idaho that I was supposed to spend some time with her, but I had already planned a trip to Yosemite and I was looking forward to being alone. I put the note in my purse and finished packing the car. In the morning, I said goodbye to Phil and the kids, and Maxx and I drove to the Sierras.

My first day in Yosemite, I awoke early, made a hot cup of tea and walked Maxx out to a small wild grass clearing. I took in a deep breath of the clear crisp air and looked up at the enormous granite walls that encircled the valley. The morning sun shining off the face of El Capitan suddenly made my life seem trivial. My years on this planet would be less than an inch of its 3,000-foot strata, and, at least for the day, that put my concerns in perspective.

I hiked over the creek and up the John Muir Trail, thinking of Anne most of the way. Did she still think of me, or was that energy now focused on somebody else? The forest was looking darker, the path getting narrower as I passed a waterfall trickling down the face of a moss-covered granite wall. What would I say if I saw her again? Would I be angry, tell her about my pain and frustration? No, none of that seemed important any more.

When the sun went down, I ate a sandwich and crawled into the van. I wrote in my journal for a few minutes then closed my eyes and went to the image of the well. My body felt clean. I had no desire to return to the cavern. Madame appeared and encouraged me to keep bathing, so I took another bath in the pool, cleansing myself under the falls, falling asleep still in the visualization.

A thunderstorm woke me in the middle of the night. Maxx jumped in my bed and began licking open my eyes.

"Okay, boy, you can sleep here, but you'd better not have fleas."

He wagged his tail and put his head down, his fur warming my side as the rhythm of the rain on the roof of the van sent me back to sleep.

In the morning, I checked with the ranger, who told me the forecast was that the storm would last for a week. I jumped back in the van and looked at Maxx.

"I guess we're supposed to go to San Luis Obispo."

I left the park and traversed the state. My older brother, James, lived in San Luis Obispo. I'd go to his place for the night and call Mary in the morning.

In the central valley, I drove past a tomato farm that went on for miles. Thinking of my brother, I leaned on the accelerator and increased my speed. James had told me he believed my memories, then became more present in my parents' lives to compensate for my absence. I was angry that he comforted them and didn't stand up for me, but James had always been the child who tried to make every-body happy and, like the rest of my family, he hadn't changed.

The high speed was arousing my body, pumping my adrenaline as I flew passed a truck on the two-lane highway. I could end it all right now, press the accelerator to the floor and wrap this van around one of those utility poles. The speedometer hit ninety and the wheels started to vibrate. Ninety-five... Ninety...

Maxx whined, and I let up on the gas. Phil would kill me if anything happened to his dog. I pulled back to seventy and put in a new C.D.

I arrived in San Luis Obispo and called my brother from a gas station.

"Hey, Dawner, where are you?"

"I'm in town. I need a place to stay for the night."

"Great! Come on over. We're having some people for dinner and we'll set an extra place."

"That's all right. All I need is a hot shower and a bed."

"You've got it."

James lived in a residential neighborhood, in a fixer-upper he and his wife were remodeling. When I pulled up to the driveway, James was waiting for me at the curb. It was hard to believe he was almost forty-years-old, a slender man with a wiry medium-height frame and curly, brown hair receding at the forehead. Through the window of my van, I could see he had aged, his tan skin beginning to look weathered. I stepped out of the van and he opened his arms.

"I was starting to think you didn't want to see me anymore," he said as he picked me up and twirled me around.

"I was mad, but I wasn't that mad."

He grabbed my bag and stopped me before I entered the house. "Hey Dawn, these guys coming over for dinner tonight, they have AIDS. One of them only has a few more months to live."

"I'm sorry."

"I just wanted to prepare you."

He opened the door and both of his grade-school-aged daughters came up and hugged me. "Aunt Dawn, Aunt Dawn." I wrapped my arms around them. I'd missed his kids, but seeing them made me miss mine all the more.

We went downstairs and I took a shower, then colored with the girls until I was called for dinner. When I walked upstairs, James introduced me to Steve and Mark. They were both in their thirties but looked well into their fifties. Mark had a nervous laugh. His body was frail but not as thin as Steve's.

I sat down next to Steve, who talked as if somebody had a loaded gun to his head, rambling incessantly about his illness as if he didn't have enough time left to make sense out of his life. He told me about the lesions on his skin, the tremors in his body and the dentist who had refused to take him as a patient. I listened with compassion. I knew the fear of death — but not the way he did.

When Mark and Steve left, James came down to my room. I sat up in bed and he straddled a chair next to me.

"Dawn, I know you're angry with me, but this has been really difficult. I love Dad, and I've always respected him as a father and a role model. This whole thing has turned me inside out."

"I didn't want to know this about him either, but, now that we do, I don't think we can pretend that it didn't happen."

"I don't pretend like it didn't happen. I confronted Dad, but he said he didn't do it and told me he never wanted to talk about it again. I don't know what else I could have done after that."

"But you told me you believed me."

He nodded. "I do, but I'll be honest with you. I don't know if I believe all your memories, but I believe some of them." A tear rolled down his face. "And... I'm so sorry. I've thought about it a million times. We lived in the same house. Why didn't I see? Why didn't I pay more attention? Why didn't I do something to help you? I'm your older brother and I should have protected you."

I had never cried in front of my family, and I didn't want to start.

"You didn't know. And even if you had, you were only a kid. You couldn't have done anything to help me."

"I'm so sorry."

"So am I."

We talked for over an hour, then James handed me an extra blanket and turned off my light. When he closed the door, I closed my eyes and went back to the well and checked through my body for the humiliating feelings of shame. But I felt surprisingly good, my soul as clean as the water in the pool.

In the morning, James came in early to say good-bye.

"I'm going to take the kids to school, then Amy and I have to go to work. Will you be around tonight?"

"I don't know. A friend of mine lives around here somewhere. I'm going to give her a call and see if we can get together."

"Okay, let me know what you're doing."

"Thanks, James." He kissed me goodbye and I curled up in bed. It was raining outside and it felt good to sleep in. I closed my eyes and the image of me sitting in my beach chair next to the well spontaneously appeared. And in front of me to the right, hovering a few feet from my chair, was the image of a large, brilliant, white light that looked like a twinkling star.

What are you? I asked with my thoughts.

The Christ light.

Green and blue light radiated from the image and through my body. My eyes flew open and I jerked up in bed.

What the hell was the Christ light?

A vibration of energy moved up my spine. My body doing something without my permission made me feel completely out of control. I jumped out of bed and ran upstairs, pacing the living room, wishing somebody was home.

"The Christ light! What does the Christ light want with me?" I grabbed a pillow and held it to my chest. "I don't need this. I really, really, don't need this."

I ran out to the van and found the note with Mary's number, grabbed Maxx and took him back into the house, and dialed the phone.

"Please answer, please answer."

"Hello." Thank God.

"Mary?"

"Yes."

"Hi, this is Dawn Kohler. I'm in town visiting my brother and I thought maybe we could get together."

"Oh, that would be wonderful. Do you have dinner plans this evening?"

"No, I don't."

She gave me directions to her home and we planned to meet at five. I hung up and made some toast, my hands shaking as I buttered it, my mouth too dry to swallow. I washed it down with a glass of water and jumped in the van with Maxx.

I drove west till I hit a beach, then got out and ran along the deserted sand. The ocean had blown out from the storm, the wind gusting so hard it felt like I was running in place. I ran for a couple of miles, then started to walk, sensations washing through me that were out of my control. Powerful sexual fantasies that took me to the brink of orgasm, then I dropped into terror, an extreme survival fear that lasted for minutes. My hearing became hypersensitive. When Maxx barked at a bird, I couldn't tell where the sound was coming from — Maxx, my mind, or the space in between.

I ran back to the van, jumped in the back and lay down to relax. As I stared out the window, my eyes clouded with a vision, an image of me reaching out to comfort several people standing on a street, translucent figures of other humans who I realized were an extension of me, all of us part of a greater organism. My chest filled with the deepest sense of self love, one that included all beings as part of who I am. Then the vision disappeared and my paranoia returned.

I stayed at the beach until a quarter to five, then loaded up Maxx and headed for Mary's house.

Her house was off a dirt road. I pulled up next to a windmill she had built to fuel her home. She came out from behind the house in a long, white shirt and a gardening hat. Her straight, gray, shoulder-length hair was thick and beautiful, and I noticed her gracefully aging body was still sturdy and strong as I hugged her hello.

"Did you have any problems finding the house?"

"No, and I'm very glad I'm here." As we walked into the kitchen, I told her about the image of the light and the flow of energy that was barreling through my body, recounting the sensations without taking a breath.

"I've had enough," I said. "Whatever is happening to me is happening too fast. I've lost all control — it's taking me over."

She poured me a hot cup of tea and stepped up to her library, where she pulled several books from her shelf and laid them on the table.

"What you're experiencing," she said, " is really quite normal for the process you're in."

"This is normal?"

She nodded. "In the base of the spine there is a coil of energy that is known in many countries as the Kundalini. When it is activated, the Kundalini energy moves through the chakras system. The sensations you felt — of losing control, of hypersensitive hearing, visions and intense sexual arousal — are reactions to the energy as it opens the chakras." Her voice deepened. "The Kundalini is powerful. If it moves through your body too quickly, it can be very damaging."

Her concern added to my fears.

"Dawn, I've been worried about you. It's not advisable to do this type of deep spiritual work without a teacher who has had firsthand experience with the process of transformation."

"I have a good therapist."

"Has she done this kind of work before?"

"No, but she's probably read about it." I put down my tea. "Mary, I need to slow this energy down. It's too much."

She stood up and reached for her purse. "Come on, I'll buy you a steak."

"A steak?"

"You need a heavy meal. A steak ought to ground you for a couple of hours."

I wasn't hungry, but I forced down a filet mignon. After a couple of bites my mind and body began to slow down.

"Mary, if the image I received really was the Christ light, why didn't I feel loved when it appeared?"

"I think the love comes when you open up and actually accept the Christ light as part of self. The blue and green light you describe probably activated the Kundalini energy. It's preparing you for the divine encounter."

"Divine encounter?"

"Yes. When you get home you can read some of the books I will give you. Most of them describe the roller-coaster sensations of the Kundalini energy as part of the spiritual transformation process, a phase that is often referred to as the *dark night of the soul*. It's the most rapid and turbulent part of the cleansing process."

"My mind feels like it's being annihilated."

"In a sense, it is, and your reaction is typical. People often want to quit at this point. But you don't want to get stuck in the Kundalini energy phase, it amplifies your longings, insecurities and fears. For the sake of your own comfort, you need to keep going."

After dinner, we went back to her house and I read through some of the books she suggested. There were many Christian, Hindu and Buddhist texts that described the Kundalini energy and the dark night of the soul. The one I picked up first was called *A Path With Heart*, written by Jack Kornfield, an American Buddhist who studied in Asia. He describes the *dark night of the soul* as a process that can take months, even years. It is a period where longings, grasping and anxiety became magnified — a cleansing process that is necessary to open to all that is and let go of all that has been.

I went to bed that night frightened and lonely. My life as I knew it was over, and in my heart, I clung with desperation to the people I loved: Philip, the kids, and Anne. My yearning to see her again was so deep and relentless that I would have faced any demon in hell if it meant I could have crawled into her arms just one more time.

Early in the morning, I packed to go home. Mary cautioned me to take it slowly.

"Ground yourself with heavy foods, routines, people that make you feel secure."

I thanked her, drove home, and enmeshed myself in the arms of my family — and a deep-dish pepperoni pizza.

On Tuesday, I started my session with Judith telling her about my trip and my experience with the Kundalini energy. As I assumed,

Judith hadn't experienced it, but she had read about it and the effects it has had on people throughout history.

"Dawn, I think I need some clarity," she said. "It's natural for the expansion of your consciousness to cause some paranoia, but it sounds like you're afraid of the Christ light."

"I am."

"Why?"

"Because it wants to talk to me."

"How do you know?"

"I've seen this light before. I saw it in an image when I first started with Anne. Back then, it looked far away, like a distant star. But now, it's right here, and it wants to talk to me."

"So, talk to it."

My hands started to sweat. "What if the Christ light tells me something I don't want to hear? What if it makes me do something I don't want to do? What if it brainwashes me? Sends me out to parties to tell people Jesus loves them? I don't want to be like that. I don't want to be a born-again Christian."

"You have some interesting associations. Do you have a Christian upbringing?"

"No, and the few times I tried to learn about Christianity, I found more confusion than comfort."

"Give me an example."

I let out a deep breath as I recalled Joyce's death. "When I was a teenager, a friend of mine died. It scared me, so I went to a couple of Christian churches looking for some understanding. But all I heard at the time was a bunch of rules, sins that kept me from being accepted into God's kingdom."

"What did they tell you?"

The dire warning about sex before marriage popped into my mind. "They told me sex before marriage was a sin. Judith, if sex before marriage is a sin, there aren't going to be a lot of people in heaven."

"How old were you when you went to that church?"

"Fourteen."

"You're fourteen-years old, you're dealing with the issue of your mortality, and a priest or minister lists sex before marriage as a sin that has the potential of keeping you from eternal life?"

"Yes."

"Dawn, although you suppressed the memories, you knew you had been raped, and I imagine when the minister informed you that sex before marriage was a sin, you probably decided you were already damned to hell."

I felt my stomach sink. Judith handed me a tissue.

"That's not all," I said. "The Christians make heaven sound like an exclusive country club, a reward for the Puritan ethic, and I just don't fit into that kind of group. It doesn't feel right to me."

"What do you think heaven is?"

"A place in our minds where we stop terrorizing ourselves."

She nodded. "And the Christ light?"

"I don't know. Do you?"

"I know that the image you described is both universal and subjective."

"What do you mean?"

"It's subjective in that, based on people's cultures and experiences, the light has been interpreted as being God, Jesus, the Buddha, Mohammed. Throughout history there have been many different names for the same experience."

"Then why did it say to me it was the Christ light?"

"Because I think your perceptions of Christ are what you need to correct. You have to let go of other people's interpretations and determine what the Christ light means to you."

"Have you had other clients experience the Christ light?"

"Yes, I have, but, like I said, it's subjective. I've heard the light called by many names."

"What happens when people experience it?"

She smiled. "They don't need to see me anymore."

I smiled back and reached for my keys.

"But, Dawn, I feel compelled to warn you. Most of what I believe you are going through is a transformation that seems to be exposing you to the awareness of a higher-self. And, there also seems to be a a universal element to your process. If you are indeed receiving some kind of direct communication from a spiritual dimension, it could be very difficult for your mind and body to absorb that kind of energy in human form. Historically, people who have had those kinds of encounters have had a difficult time assimilating them."

I stared at her but didn't respond. Her warning frightened me, as if I was the cowardly lion about to enter the great cathedral of Oz.

"Have you written Anne's eulogy yet?" she asked as I walked towards the door.

"Judith, I really don't want to do that."

"I know you don't, but you have been denied many rites of passage in your life, and you need to recognize and write about them so your mind can assimilate the change in you — and in your relationship with Anne."

"I don't know if I can."

"It's time. I want Anne's eulogy by our next session."

The storm in Yosemite had followed me south. It was raining when I came home from Judith's office. Our three-car garage no longer had room for a car. Phil's pool table took up half the room and he'd converted the other half into his new office. I jumped out into the rain and slipped through the side door. Maxx was lying under the pool table. Phil was building a mud volcano with Michael.

"How was your session?" he asked.

"Oh, fine." I thought about telling him about the Christ light, but decided I might want to wait until I knew what it meant.

"My flight leaves at eight o'clock tomorrow," he said. "Can you give me a ride to the airport?"

It took me a minute to remember where he was going. My brother-in-law was on his last tour in the Navy, and as part of the shake-down from long deployment, the men could invite a relative to join the last leg of the voyage. Phil was flying to Hawaii, then sailing home on a destroyer.

"Sure, I'll take you," I said. I went up to the nest and pulled out my journal. What did the Christ light mean? Was it God? Was it Jesus? Did it matter?

I put down my pen and recalled my chance meeting with Susan Wells in the bookstore, and my reading with her in her home. She was the only person I knew who looked as though she had experienced the light. Everything about her seemed to exude clarity and love. I called her that night and made an appointment.

Susan smiled warmly as I entered her home. She offered me some tea as we sat on the white chenille couches in her small, white-carpeted living room.

"What can I do for you?" she asked.

I explained the cleaning process that I had been experiencing and the vision of the light. "Do you know what the light is?"

"I see it as a kind of transformer," she said. "It connects us to the energy of God so that we can absorb it in human form."

"Has this ever happened to you?

"Yes, several times. It's a very gentle and beautiful experience. It provides a bath of white light that rejuvenates you with a sense of love."

"Then why am I so afraid?"

She looked at me as though she was looking through me. "You were abused, weren't you?"

"Yes."

"By your father?"

"Yes." It was still difficult to admit.

"Dawn, a spiritual awakening for a child of dysfunction can be very frightening. The end of this process requires total trust, faith and surrender. It's the only way you can accept and embody who you really are."

"I have to surrender to the Christ light?"

"You have to let go of your resistance in order to experience the divine love and wholeness the light has to offer."

"I don't want to let go of my resistance to something bigger than me. I'm afraid I'm going to be hurt." I looked up at the ceiling, trying to hold back a tear.

"Dawn, the Christ light is not your human father. It's a gift, and it's here to love you. And if you're still afraid, you can always make a deal with it. Set up the conditions in which it can enter."

"What do you mean?"

"Ask the Christ light for an act of love. Let it prove itself to you."

"You can do that?"

"Sure. It's not like you can piss off the Christ light. It's here to help you. Ask and you will receive. If it's in your best interest, you'll get what you want."

She handed me a tissue and Anne's eulogy came to mind.

"Susan, there's another thing that's been bothering me. My therapist has been trying to get me to write this person's eulogy — Anne, the woman who helped me get started on this journey. But, when I think about writing it, it doesn't feel right. I understand that my therapist wants me to give the relationship closure, but the finality of a eulogy seems to cut too deep. She's at my core, and it doesn't feel right to try and destroy it, or leave it behind."

"What's Anne's full name?"

"Anne Myers"

She closed her eyes and went into trance. A moment later, she looked as though she was basking in a pleasurable experience. "This is a very loving relationship," she said. "In fact, it goes beyond love, it has to do with your original creation. She paused as if hearing something. "You're part of the same energy," she said. "Your spiritual DNA is identical. It would be impossible to give her up on a spiritual level." She focused her eyes back on me. "But your therapist is right. You will need to give her up on the physical plane. You're not going to see Anne again in this lifetime."

The stab was that of a sudden death; tears poured down my face.

"Then, that's what I want," I said. "If I can ask the Christ light to show me an act of love, then I want that act of love to be to see Anne again."

"Dawn, you don't want to try and change destiny."

My voice cracked. "Susan, the last time I saw her I was in so much pain I couldn't feel her love. I couldn't feel the hug she gave me when she said good-bye, and I want that moment back. I want to be able to feel what we shared. I want to know it was real."

"Then envision her in your mind and ask for a phone call."

"I don't want a phone call," I cried. "I want to see her again."

"Dawn, I could be wrong, but I don't think that's going to happen."

I took a sobering breath. It was unlikely that even the Christ light could make Anne suddenly appear in my life.

"All right. I'll ask for the phone call."

Susan offered me another tissue as she walked me out the door. "How's your book coming?"

"I'm just waiting for the ending."

I went out and sat in the car. Closing my eyes, I prayed to the light: *For an act of love, can I please, please talk to Anne.* I let my thoughts go.

Three days.

In three days, it would be Sunday.

Confident that the Christ light wouldn't let me down, I went into the weekend in a better mood than usual. Philip was still in Hawaii. I stayed busy taking the kids to birthday parties and soccer games. Sunday arrived in no time, and when I awoke, I was full of faith, sure that Anne would call and I would finally get a chance to resolve our relationship—to find out what was real, not by her words, but by the tone in her voice.

I got out of bed, the possibilities of the day running through my mind like a high-speed chase. Maybe Anne was in town. Maybe I would get to see her. Or maybe she would call from overseas. What if she called collect? What if she called collect and the kids answered? And what about the phone? What if it wasn't working when she called? I knew I was being neurotic, but that didn't stop me from checking the receiver and telling the kids to let me answer the phone if it rang.

By noon, the phone hadn't rung and the thoughts that began darting through my head were more anxious, less optimistic. Maybe hearing from Anne was too much to ask.

I didn't want to leave the house and miss the call, so the kids and I went out in the yard. I dug up weeds while they made mud cakes. By three o'clock my yard looked like hell and my hopes of hearing from Anne were rapidly dissolving. Was this a set-up for another lesson? Or had everything that had happened to me over the past two and half years been one remarkable series of meaningless coincidences?

I made the kids dinner. This had nothing to do with Anne anymore — this was a stand-off between me and the Christ light. If God existed, she'd call.

By the time I put the kids to bed, I hated myself. The light was here to offer me love, and I had tried to cut a deal with it. Maybe Susan was wrong. Maybe you could *piss off* the Christ light and maybe that's exactly what I had done. Should I drop to my knees and pray for forgiveness? Or should I...

The phone rang. I ran to my room. Where was the cordless? I threw the pillow off my bed. The third ring. It was in the bathroom. I rushed across the room and picked it up from the counter.

"Hello."

"Hi, Dawn, is Phil there?"

"Oh...hi, Jon. No, he won't be home until Wednesday."

"You sound so happy to hear from me," he said.

"I'm sorry, I've just had a bad day."

We talked for a minute and hung up. I needed to get some food in me. This dark night of the soul was turning me into a nut case. I went downstairs and fixed myself a peanut butter and jelly sandwich. Sucking the jelly out from in between the bread, I thought of the worst possibility of all. What if my parents were right? What if two years of psychotherapy had made me psychotic?

I went up to my bed and closed my eyes. *Be patient.*

By 9:30 my hopes had all but faded. I was lost, abandoned again by Anne, abandoned again by God. I crawled into bed, curled up in the sheets and again, cried myself to sleep.

In the morning, my thoughts were clearer, and I realized upon waking that my prayer had been answered. The answer was no. It wasn't in my best interest to hear from Anne. Humbled by my childish attempts to control my destiny, I got up and went on with my day.

That night, I put the kids to bed and retreated to my desk. The only door left was the one I didn't want to open, the one that said write Anne's eulogy. I turned on the computer, sat back in my chair, closed my eyes and imagined myself at the foot of her grave. It was a simple plot marked by a small, brass plate under an oak tree on a hill covered with wildflowers. I focused on the plate and the inscription appeared: *I don't judge you. I just love you.*

I opened my eyes and began to write.

Anne's Eulogy

Anne,

> *You came into my life when an early death was the only path I was on. In a matter of months, you opened your heart to mine and gave me a love that kept me alive. You gave me a love that made me feel like I belonged in the world, not for the roles I played, but for who I was.*
>
> *Over the course of the next year, you became a loving therapist, friend, mentor and a part of my family, the part that was missing. Your gentle wisdom and caring soul gave me the strength to open the doors to mine. You gave me the courage to feel the pain of an ugly past and showed me the light to a joyous future. You taught me, you believed in me, and you gave me hope. But above all else, you gave me a safe place to be held. And for the first time in my life, I could hand my power over to somebody else, and not be hurt by it, but nurtured.*

May you rest in peace.
God bless you
Amen

I finished the eulogy and closed my eyes. In my mind, I dropped to my knees and sobbed at the foot of her grave. The pain of letting her go left a void in my entire being.

The next day, I surrendered it to Judith.

"Here it is," I said, tossing it to her.

"Good. Now read it to me."

I stared at her in protest.

"Go ahead, Dawn, read it."

I sat down in my chair and began. When I finished we were both in tears.

"Judith, it hurts in every cell of my body."

She reached for her glasses and asked to see the eulogy. When she was finished reading it, she handed it back.

"I want you to read this again, but this time replace Anne's name with yours and put it in the first person."

I picked up the eulogy and read it out loud.

Dawn's eulogy

Dawn,

> *You came into my life when an early death was the only path I was on. In a matter of months, you opened your heart to me and gave me a love that kept me alive. You gave me a love that made me feel like I belonged in the world, not for the roles I played, but for who I was.*
>
> *Over the course of the next year, you became a loving therapist, friend, mentor and a part of my family, the part that was missing. Your gentle wisdom and caring soul gave me the strength to open the doors to myself. You gave me the courage to feel the pain of an ugly past and you showed me the light to a joyous future. You taught me, you believed in me, and you gave me hope. But above all else, you gave me a safe place to be held. And for the first time in my life, I could feel my power with somebody else and not be hurt, but nurtured.*

I looked up at Judith. "This eulogy is about me," I said.

"That's how I hear it. And I think that's why it hurts in every cell of your body."

"Then why can't I feel this love when I think of me?"

"Because you have projected your love onto Anne. The love, understanding, and knowledge you were able to obtain in your relationship with her was really your own. You felt it, and it was your experience."

"But, I wasn't in this alone."

"No, you weren't, but your experience of it was your own. That's how we learn. You felt understood and Anne showed you what that looked like. She expressed it and you labeled it. This is understanding. This is what understanding looks like. But the understanding came from you, for you. And that's also true for the love, compassion and wisdom that you felt. She showed you what it looked like, but you felt it. It was your own experience."

I didn't like what I was hearing. It sounded like I was in this love alone.

"It sounds so cold," I said. "Anne was the love object and everything between us was my own projection? A wall that I spewed my emotions on?"

"Dawn, I don't know how Anne experienced you, but I don't think it matters."

"It matters to me. When my heart connects with somebody, I want to trust that it was real and not just a bunch of transferences, counter-transferences and projections."

"It was real. It was your experience, and our feelings and experiences are always real."

I ran my fingers through the top of my hair. "Judith, I don't think you get it, and, to tell the truth, I'm not sure I do. But there was more to my relationship with Anne than I can translate into words, or you can identify by a theory."

"I believe that's true, but I also believe that the love you feel for Anne is the love you have for yourself. All you have to do is own it."

Own it. How was I supposed to own it? I felt faceless. I could see it in Anne, but not in myself.

I reached out to Phil and the kids, hoping to squeeze some kind of loving sensation from my chest, but there was nothing there. I was shut down and all I could do was pretend. Pretend to be happy while we played at the park, smile through my frustration when Phil kissed me goodnight. It was if I was in a world where I didn't belong, searching for a heart I wasn't sure I had.

I continued to go down to the beach and take Tai Chi lessons from Russ. My postures with the Twelve Hands were becoming lethargic. I now swayed between screaming in frustration and collapsing from exhaustion. Russ appeared amused with my struggle.

"Don't fight your frustration. Work with it."

"How do I do that?"

"Stay after class and I'll show you."

The other women went home; it was cloudy and cold and, except for Russ and me, the beach was deserted. Russ demonstrated a Yoga exercise designed to open the heart chakra. I followed, pushing the bottom of my palms and the tips of my fingers together as I pressed my thumbs against my chest. With my fingers pointed in front of me, I extended my arms toward the ocean and then again back to my sternum.

"Push harder," he commanded. "And move your arms slowly."

"How long do I have to do this?"

"Till you're finished."

Twenty minutes into the exercise, a wave of energy came up from my center and into my chest, a sensation of warm liquid that released me from both frustration and fatigue.

Russ looked into my eyes. "I think we found life."

For the rest of the day, I was calm and more present with my children. I nursed the warmth in my chest by drinking hot tea thoughout the day and sank into a warm bath that night to release myself even further. At 9:00 o'clock, I melted into bed and a few hours later, I found myself in one of the most vivid dreams I had ever experienced.

In the dream, I walked out of a dark, cold night into the small, beige-carpeted condominium I had purchased in college. I was wearing jeans, my hands in the pockets of a long, navy-blue, down jacket that warmed the chill that had permeated my skin. On a daybed in the living room sat Anne, wearing a soft pink sweater that extended to her ankles. A woman in her late fifties stood a few feet away. She had the medium round build of my mother, short, sassy salt-and-pepper hair, and harsh, black eyeliner that accentuated her pale skin and bitter eyes.

I locked eyes with Anne. Her soul was illuminated, her love much stronger than I had felt in real life. I walked toward her cautiously.

"They told me I was never going to see you again," I said.

She smiled and slowly shook her head. "No, Dawn, that's not true."

Tears of relief rolled down my cheeks as I dropped to my knees and collapsed in her lap. The touch of her body made me feel as if I had safely arrived home from a terrifying battle.

Anne placed her arm inside the back of my jacket and lightly pressed down on my last three vertebrae. The pressure on my spine released a wave of warm energy that rolled up my back, through the top of my head, and back down the front of my body. My chest flooded with wholeness. My soul was finally at peace.

"Get off of her!" The older woman who had a strong southern accent, grabbed me by the jacket, yanked me off of Anne and threw me against the door. "Get out of here!"

My body felt like a shell, as if the woman had just torn me from the pulse of my own heart.

The woman pointed at me and laughed. "She's been a fool over you!" she said to Anne. "She's sick, dependent, enmeshed, obsessed!"

I stood paralyzed in the doorway.

"You were her therapist," the woman told Anne. "And you have no business in her life. I don't want you to see her again, ever!"She grabbed Anne by the hand and took her up a staircase, ridiculing me as she walked, convincing Anne to stay away. I watched in humility as they walked away, longing for Anne to turn around, desperate to be back in the safety of her arms.

"Get out of here!" the woman yelled again, as I dissolved into a shame over the intensity of my love for Anne and bolted out the door in hopes I'd never be seen again.

I ran out into the night, down a dark, narrow path and onto a road in La Jolla. I couldn't escape fast enough, so I dove into the air, using all my strength to propel myself forward using frantic swimming motions. At the top of the road was a bright-red stop light. The Catholic church was on one side, my elementary school on the other. My intention was to run the light, but then I heard a child's cry.

I awoke trembling and gasping for air, the sheets soaked with my sweat. Another cry. It was my daughter, Erica. I jumped out of bed and ran to her room. But by the time I reached her, she had fallen back to sleep.

I stumbled into the bathroom, got a drink of water, splashed a little on my face, then went to lie down in the nest. *Please help me, God. What do I do next?*

In the morning, I awoke to an image of the light, and a chanting in my mind, a gentle rhythm that sounded like background music in an elevator.

Love her with all your heart, with all your mind, and with all your soul.
It was about Anne. I repeated the message and burst into tears, finally receiving permission to do what my heart desired — to return to the wholeness I felt in Anne's arms. I was to love her with all my heart, with all my mind, and with all my soul.

I walked into my next therapy session and quickly shut the door, feeling the anger shooting out of my eyes as I told Judith about the dream and the message I received that morning.

"In all the time that Anne's been gone," I said, "I have tried to find understanding through friends, therapists, and support groups. And never, not once, has anybody ever said to me, 'Why don't you just love her?' "

Judith was speechless.

"It's so damn simple."

I threw myself into the chair. "Do you know, it's been more humiliating telling people that I fell in love with a woman therapist than it has been telling them I was raped by my father? That's sick, Judith. That's really sick."

Judith nodded. "I'm sorry, Dawn, and you have all the right in the world to be angry."

Neither one of us spoke for several minutes.

"Can you tell me more about the woman in your dream? The one who pulled you off of Anne."

"She was a bitch. A bitter, abrasive, condescending bitch."

"And who in your life do you think she represents?"

"I don't know. She laughed at me like my mother, but the ridicule felt like it was coming from society — the popular belief, or the latest therapeutic theory."

"And do I represent that to you?" she asked.

"Sometimes."

She looked hurt, as if she had taken my words deeply to heart. "Close your eyes."

"You're really pushing it," I said.

"I know, but please do it anyway."

Why I obeyed her was beyond me. I closed my eyes and sat back in my chair.

"Bring back into your awareness the scene from the dream where the woman pulled you off of Anne. When you have her in your mind, I want you to become her. Take on her consciousness."

As I centered my mind in the image of the woman, a subtle pain began to fill the emptiness in my chest. I was surprised at the tenderness behind her veneer. "She's a very hurt person. She's been judged harshly and from her pain she does the same." The energy in my chest continued to swell, coming from my center, as if I had just connected through an umbilical cord to a large pool of world-wide suffering.

"This pain I feel, it's big... much bigger than me. It feels like it is coming from the center of the earth." The anguish felt as though it was inflating my body. My voice rose as the words rolled off my tongue." We don't understand who we are, our relationships to each other. When we judge our love — when we judge ourselves, we are tearing our souls apart." The pain was universal, a heart being ignorantly destroyed by its own organism. My back arched from the energy, and my chest felt as though it was about to burst.

"Dawn, bring in Elisa or Madame to help you. There's too much energy here. Ask them what you need to do with it."

Madame appeared.

Write about it.

"She says to write about it. We have to stop hurting ourselves. The judgments are destroying us."

The painful energy began to subside as I opened my eyes and caught my breath. "That was wild."

"Madame is a universal figure. You're tapping into collective consciousness. That can be very powerful."

"It's very painful. It's the same pain I felt in the dream when I was pulled away from Anne, but it's deeper. Much deeper."

Judith leaned forward. "What did Anne represent to you in the dream?"

"My heart. My soul. There was something I saw in her that was me. I can't explain it, Judith, but it was more than a projection. It was something very real."

"Projections are real."

"Yes, but it wasn't just in my mind. It was also in hers."

I wanted to be validated, but Judith's face was expressionless.

"I want you to go home and write more about the dream. Go into Anne's consciousness, the other woman's, and then back into yours. Write it like a play and describe each character. They all represent a part of you, and we want to try and understand them."

Her words went through me. "Judith, I'm supposed to love Anne with all my heart, all my mind and all my soul. That's a lot of energy to put into somebody who might not care if I still exist."

"Dawn, it doesn't matter how Anne feels. This is about you."

I picked up my keys.

"It matters a lot to me how Anne feels," I said. "I want to believe that I connected to something other than myself."

"I think you have."

Chapter 12

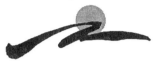

The more I tried to love Anne, the more I started to hate her. The woman had abandoned me, left me in a hospital without following up. She never responded to my letter or gave me a chance for a closure. How could I love her? I wasn't sure I even liked her.

I sat in bed looking at the clock. It was 6:00 am and I still had time to run to the beach before Phil and the kids woke up for breakfast. I quietly put on my sweats and hit the trail, the pace of my stride faster than normal as I continued to think about Anne. Was this some kind of irritating lesson on forgiveness? And if it was, how would I rise to the occasion? How was I going to love Anne with all my heart, soul and mind when doing so made me want to track her down, tie her to a tree, and place a noose around her neck, tightening it until she could barely breathe.

By the time I reached the beach, I had settled down. I stood in the sand for a moment and watched the blue-gray waters churning under the influence of a full-moon tide. The face of the sea was turbulent; the depth had little clarity. If I could only understand Anne, talk to her and find out what she was thinking. There had to be a good reason for all this — probably something I'd done. Maybe it was that phone call I'd made to her after my massage with Joanne.

I came home to the smell of pancakes. Philip tossed them on the griddle while I made the lunches for the kids.

"Why did you ditch me last night?" he said.

I was so used to waking up in the nest, I'd forgotten how I got there. "I was hot."

"You always say that."

"I get hot a lot."

I was looking forward to my afternoon session with Judith. The boundary around her tall slender body, the strong poise that once would have been threatening to me, was now a comfort. And I found myself appreciating how healing it was to be in a relationship that had such clarity.

"I think I understand why Anne decided to cut off contact with me," I told Judith as I sat down in our next session.

"This ought to be good," she said.

"A couple of days before Anne left, I had a massage from a woman Anne knew. She told me that Anne had always known she was leaving, and I jumped to the conclusion that Anne hadn't been honest with me. I called Anne to ask her about it, and I think when she heard how out of my mind I was, it scared her away."

"You scared Anne?"

"Yes."

"So, this is all your fault."

"Basically, yes."

"And if this is all your fault, then you can forgive Anne and go back to loving her with all your heart, soul, and mind?"

I could feel myself shrinking. "Well, that's what I had in mind."

"Let me see if I have this right. Your father abused you, because you needed to be punished. Your mother neglected you, because you pushed her away. And Anne left you without closure or a consistent means of communication, because you scared her by exposing your vulnerability."

"It sounds different when you say it."

"Dawn, you're not responsible for their neglect."

"But it's the only way I can make sense out of their actions."

"You can't make sense out of the senseless."

"Then how can I forgive her?"

"Forgiveness is overrated."

"It is?"

"Yes. I don't even think it's necessary."

"But can there be love without forgiveness?" I asked

"There can be love despite forgiveness."

I shook my head. Why didn't this path come with better instructions?

"Judith, if I could just talk to Anne, I know I could work this out and come to terms with it."

"Or, you could put your energy into another direction."

"What's that?"

"Anne isn't in your life, but Philip is. You might be better off if you focused your love on him."

I sighed. She didn't understand. "I know this path sounds ridiculous to you, but I trust my messages. I trust that when I see Anne's soul, I will see my own, and I believe that in order to do that, I have to love her with all my heart, soul and mind. And, to tell you the truth, I don't understand why the focus is on Anne, but I know that it is. And I believe that if I can get my heart open through my relationship with her, it will be open for Philip."

She nodded. "Okay, then can you accept Anne for all her human fallibility's and love her anyway?"

"If I could trust her intentions were loving."

"So, if Anne's not trustworthy, then she's not worthy of being loved."

"Don't confuse me."

"Just doing my job." She smiled. "It might help you to understand that there is no such thing as unconditional trust."

"There isn't?"

"No. There are things you can trust that people will do. And there are things that you can trust that people will not do. And within both, there is a margin of error."

"Are you trying to tell me my expectations are too high?"

"Maybe. Give me three things that you trust about me."

I looked at her. "I trust that you will show up for our appointments. That you will stay focused on our conversations, and that you will not leave my emotional state for your own."

"Okay. I will agree with you that most of the time I can be trusted for those things, but I will also tell you that, while it is rare, I have forgotten appointments. I have also become confused in therapy and lost my focus. And if I'm having a really, really bad day, I am capable of withdrawing my attention from your emotional state to take care of my own."

"You are?"

"Yes, I am. And if you are still looking for the one person who is never going to let you down, you will continue to create a setup for failure for yourself and for the person you're trying to trust."

I looked at the floor. I had set up many people and every one of them had failed.

"How do I change my expectations? Most of the time I don't even know I'm setting them up."

"You become aware of the times when your expectations are beyond the reality of our humanness, and then you re-label people's actions."

"To what?"

"To define their actions as human instead of untrustworthy."

I felt humbled by her wisdom, nodded in agreement and picked up my keys to leave. As I walked out to my car, I thought about the session. I probably had set up Anne, but it shouldn't have been beyond her humanness to give me an adequate closure, and I wasn't so enlightened as to love her with all my heart, soul and mind without also wanting to find a way to understand her motives.

That night, after putting the kids to bed, I went to the nest and turned on my computer, closed my eyes and went back to Anne's grave. This time the image felt good; the therapist was dead and I was free to talk to the gentle spirit that intermittently shone through her personality. I opened my eyes and started to type.

Why did you leave me the way you did? Why did this happen to me?

Energy bubbled in my chest before I could finish the question. I regurgitated the answer like a stream of automatic writing.

I never left you. I've been right here the entire time. But for you to find me for good, you have to stop looking in the world you see. It's an obstacle, a mirror reflection. If you want to find me for good, you have to go through your heart. When you realize where I am and you come home to my arms, there will be no separation. Your pain will be over.

I was astonished as the energy continued to steam up from my center, run down my arms and express itself through a burst of more writing.

I know it's been difficult. But I've given you everything you needed to make your way back. I have lit the path to your destination and I've held a vigil praying that you would arrive safely.

I sat back in my chair as the energy subsided. My relationship with Anne was beyond our humanness. My love for Anne was clearing the way for God.

The Christmas lights went up and the mornings grew brisker. I decorated the house with poinsettias and lined the staircase with garlands, trying to stay busy so the holiday blues wouldn't add to my depression.

I told myself it would be better this year: the pain of losing my parents wouldn't be as great, and the childhood memories wouldn't bring up the menacing fears. But something was still bothering me, and each day closer to Christmas, my chest became a little heavier. I accelerated my pace, keeping myself busy with shopping and parties, reverting to old behavior patterns as I tried to avoid the mounting depression. But two days before Christmas, my body had its say, sentencing me to bed with the flu and a 102-degree fever.

The kids tried to cheer me up with the afternoon mail, but as I flipped through the Christmas cards, I found myself feeling worse. I pulled the covers over my head and curled up in a ball. When I closed my eyes, the gold ring spontaneously appeared, the same gold ring Anne had asked me to imagine in our first guided imagery session. Inside the ring was the five-year-old child, her face glum, her shoulders drooping.

I imaged myself as an adult and sat next to her in the ring.

What's wrong? I asked.

It's Christmas, she replied. *Why can't we just hear from her at Christmas?*

I winced at her pain; after all this time, this child inside of me still believed Anne was her mother.

I'm sorry, I said to the child. But Anne's not your mother, and you can't expect her to act like one. The scab had been ripped open and the wound was oozing.

But how do I know if she's okay? How do I know if she's safe...if she's happy?"

I put the child in my lap.

You trust. You trust that the people we love are living out their lives according to what is best for them. Everybody is being taken care of by the same powers that are taking care of us. Anne is always going to be all right.

I pulled my pillow to my chest as if I was holding the child, trying to give her comfort, trying to ease the pain of breaking my own heart.

I felt well enough on Christmas day to put on a performance for the kids. They awoke at a quarter to five, and by six-thirty the first toy had been broken. Phil and I spent the morning putting together the new playhouses, sticking the batteries in the electric toys and losing every game of UNO to our three-year-old daughter, Erica.

At noon, my sister Kristen and her husband arrived. It was the first time in three years I had spent Christmas with a relative, and having them over seemed to bring some normalcy back to the occasion. I served dinner and we opened more presents; friends came over for dessert and we opened presents again. When the last person had left, Phil and I walked into our room and found the best gift of the day: our three children wrapped up in blankets like cherubs, asleep at the foot of our bed.

We carried them to their rooms and lit the fire. Phil picked up a new book and started to read. I collected the books I'd received and started to browse through the pile. The second one on the stack was an unlikely candidate: *The Tibetan Book of the Living and Dying*. A close friend had given it to me, and it surprised me that, in all the things she and I had discussed, I had never mentioned that I didn't read books that have "dead," "death," or "dying" in their titles.

I tossed it down, then noticed the yellow and orange fire reflecting off the tight cellophane cover. The least I could do was take off the wrapper. I picked up the book, and used my fingernail to pierce through the cellophane seal. Suddenly, there was a sharp pop from the air pressure and a clean light air seemed to rise from the book, surrounding me in an aura of joy. My heart warmed as it had the day Russ helped me open my heart chakra at the beach, and I felt as though I had just fallen in love — with the book.

The joy continued to rise from my warming heart, filling me with the pure elation of a child awaking to gifts on Christmas day. My fatigue had disappeared and I felt fresh and renewed as I opened the cover and began to read. In the ninth chapter, I found my message:

> *When we have prayed and aspired and hungered for the truth for a long time, for many, many lives, and when our karma has become sufficiently purified, a kind of miracle takes place. And this miracle, if we can understand and use it, can lead to the ending of ignorance forever: The inner teacher, who has been with us always, manifests in the form of the "Outer teacher," whom, almost as if by magic, we actually encounter. This encounter is the most important of any lifetime.*

> *Who is the teacher? None other than the embodiment and voice and representative of our inner teacher. The master whose human shape and human voice and wisdom we come to love with a love deeper than any other in our lives is none other than the external manifestation of the mystery*

> *of our own inner truth. What else could explain why we feel*
> *so strongly connected to him or her?*

I continued to read. For thousands of years, it had been a Tibetan practice to place a student with a teacher until the student saw his own soul in the eyes of the teacher. The divine reflection was considered to be the nature of the mind, the Buddha, the Christ within, the divine spark of our own soul.

I couldn't believe what I was reading or the elation that came with it. I looked for a passage that would describe how the student went about seeing the soul of the teacher. The blessing was usually given to the student from the teacher in person. But, if the teacher was not present with the student, the authors suggested reflecting on a picture.

I jumped out of bed and walked to the nest to take out Anne's picture, awe struck that 18 months ago she was moved to give it to me, knowing she had no idea that I would need it to reflect my soul. I sat down at my desk and pulled out the photograph. It felt good to see her face. My capacity to love her was so much greater than when she'd left.

I brought the *Tibetan book of the Living and Dying* in to my next appointment with Judith. I was talking fast, lit up with enthusiasm as I explained the experience I had when I opened the book and the passage about the Tibetan practice. Judith put on her glasses and read the passages, her reaction as dry as the arrant winter air that surrounded her office.

"From a psychological perspective," she said, "this sounds like a projection. When your mind is ready, you project your own compassion or Christ-like nature onto somebody else."

"Then how come I didn't project it onto you, or Karen, or anybody else in my life?"

"I think Anne was just the first person you trusted."

She handed me back the book and I tossed it on the table. "You really know how to suck the grace right out of this."

"I'm sorry, but I believe there are a range of people you could have had the same experience with."

"So, if I had met you first, I would have had this experience with you?"

"It would have been a different path, but I believe it would have taken you to the same place."

I shook my head. "Judith, God came to me through Anne. That's a miracle."

"That's what you take from this book?"

"From the book and from my message: *We don't really know who people are.*"

"Do you think Anne is God?"

"No, but I think God came through her, and that's why I love her so deeply."

"But she's also a human being who walks the face of this earth. She has her own problems and issues just like everyone else."

"Believe me, I know, and I'm sober about this. Anne has qualities that I feel are stronger than mine, but I have many qualities that I feel are stronger than hers. Judith, I'm not supposed to worship her. I'm just supposed to love her."

Judith asked to see the book again and opened to the passage I had read to her.

"Dawn, the teacher they refer to in this book is an enlightened master. I think Anne has the potential to be enlightened, but I do not consider her to have been at that level of consciousness when she left here."

"Neither do I, but I see something in her that goes beyond her personality."

She looked down at the book again and shook her head. "I knew Anne fairly well, and when I read this I have to wonder, which one of you is the teacher, and which one of you is the student."

"I haven't looked at it that way. But the setup when we started was that she was the teacher."

"Well, I wouldn't get hung up in that setup, especially at the rate that you process."

"Judith, I don't think that's the point. Her picture connects me to my own higher consciousness or Christ-like nature, and to get closer to it, I'm to focus on her."

"But according to this book, the practice only works if the person you are using as a mirror is an enlightened master."

"Then why did I have that reaction to the book? I was filled with love before I even opened it. And what about Anne's picture? Giving a client a picture is a highly unusual gesture, and I think it's a pretty powerful coincidence."

Her expression remained skeptical.

"Do you think Anne is conscious of any of this?"

"No, I'm sure she's not, but something moves her. She had no idea why she was giving me that picture, but it was important to her that I have it."

She shrugged. "Well, I don't see where looking at her picture is going to hurt you. You might as well give it a try." Her lack of conviction was frustrating. I wanted Judith to believe in Anne as much as I needed to, but that wasn't going to happen; boom or bust, I was on this path alone.

I went back home and finished reading the book. To receive the blessing, the faith in the light entity has to be complete. I had to trust, love and believe with all my heart that what I saw in Anne was real.

For ten minutes a day I looked at her photo, and my path, once turbulent, was now an exorcism. My dreams were drenched with emotions: the horror of drowned children, the loss of control to a fatal disease. I dreamt of Anne leaving me with the apathy of a stranger. Hours later, I dreamt of forcing my father at gunpoint to admit to my family what he had done to me. I awoke in sweats, tremors and rages, then fell back asleep and experienced another nightmare.

By that spring, I had arrived at a new state of emptiness, lost, with few chores to ground me. Phil, needing to feel productive, had taken over the tasks that had helped connect me to my life. He picked up the kids from school and planned their after-school activities, helped them with their homework and bought presents for their friends' birthday parties.

I complained one night at dinner that he was rendering me useless.

He cracked open a beer. "You just concentrate on getting better."

The nightmares continued. For two weeks I had several versions of the same dream: I stood in the living room of my childhood home as terror bellowed like smoke from the hallway. I ran out screaming into the night, waking up in a sweat and staying awake for hours.

Judith and I had talked about this particular dream before, as I remembered having had it throughout most of my life.

"When is the last time you had the nightmare?" she asked in our next session.

"Two nights ago, but the beginning of it was kind of strange."

"What was strange about it?"

I started to laugh. "I was standing at the kitchen counter listening to two lawyers, adversaries who were debating a murder trial. When they noticed it was dark outside they decided to leave. I followed then to the front door trying to convince them to stay, but they wouldn't. When they left, I walked back toward the kitchen, and when I passed the hall, this terror came over me. I ran out of the house and woke up screaming.

"What a great metaphor."

"For what?"

"Two lawyers trying to prove two separate perceptions of the truth?"

"Yes? So what does that mean?"

"I think it means your reality has been on trial. When your opposing perceptions are fighting, you're safe. You're protected from the truth. The fear doesn't set in until you're alone in the house and the fighting is over."

I felt sick to my stomach. There was still a piece of me left in that three-bedroom, stucco and shake-roof 60's-style home. I took a deep breath, "Let's do a guided imagery," I said.

"You want to go back in the nightmare?"

"No. I'm afraid I'll lose my mind if I go back into that nightmare. But I don't have a choice. That house is in my way.

"Dawn, you always have a choice."

"Yes. And I choose not to live in fear."

Judith nodded. "All right, but I'm not letting you go back into the house as a child. I want you to remain an adult the entire time, and to make sure you do, I want to start in the garden."

I closed my eyes and imagined the garden. The garden, which had formerly appeared inside my forehead, now appeared over my heart. The grounds were spacious and light, the tall bushes and dark forest that once enclosed the yard were gone, and the white bench now stood on an open bluff that looked out on a sprawling valley of yellow wheat grass and rolling, green hills.

"When you get to the garden, I want you to call up any children that are still with you." The five-year-old appeared, her face looking more like a child, trusting, tender and innocent. "Ask her who she wants to stay with her while you go back to your home in La Jolla."

Anne.

I brought in an image of Anne, a scene that came alive with vivid color as Anne knelt and opened her arms and the child ran into her warm embrace. When the five-year-old was safe, Judith told me to leave the garden and go back into the dream. I focused my consciousness on the entrance to my childhood home; taking a deep breath, I opened the front door.

The house was dark and stuffy, the windows and doors looked like they had been closed for decades. I walked passed the musty chenille couches, opening the curtains and airing out the room.

"Where are you?" Judith asked.

"I'm in the living room, looking down the hall. It's dark and narrow. I'm starting to feel the terror."

"Take a few, deep breaths and take something with you. You don't have to go down that hall by yourself."

A large, metal baseball bat appeared in my hands. I slowly walked down the hall and turned into the bathroom, flipped on the light and noticed the shower curtain was closed. I clutched my bat and flung open the plastic.

"Oh, God," I moaned.

"What's happening?" Judith asked.

"There's a red bloodstained ring around the tub. It's my blood. I have to get it off." I started to pant as I rushed to the cabinet under the sink to look for some cleanser. I swung open the doors, and a hand, severed at the wrist, rolled out of the cabinet. I started to cry.

"Judith, my hand. My right hand...my writing hand. It's under the sink."

"Do you need to put the hand back on?" she asked.

"No. I just had to see where it's been. I have to keep going. I have to leave the blood stain and the hand and keep going."

I left the bathroom and crossed the hall. It was the door to my childhood bedroom. I took a deep breath and opened it slowly. The room was dark and smelled like a musty cellar. As the image came into focus, I saw the two twin beds on each side of a white wood dresser. Above my bed, hovering like ghosts, were my father's friends, laughing at me like a trio of pirates. I grabbed my bat and ran to the window, swung open the curtains and smashed the glass. A light beamed in.

"Judith, the light's here." A blanket of brilliant, white light covered the house, shone through the window and sucked out the men. My body started to tremble. "The men are gone," I said through a heavy breath. "I have to keep going." I went back to the hall and turned left to my parents' room. I opened the door and saw the ghost of my father chained naked to his bed.

He laughed at me. "It's only a game," he said.

I jumped on his bed and started to strangle him. "I don't have to do this anymore. I never have to do this again."

"Dawn, open the window — have the light take him away."

"No...no." My emotions lost their clarity. I was whirling in feelings of terror and security.

"When he was home, I was safer. He protected the house...when he was home, he was the only one who could hurt me."

"You knew what to fear," Judith said.

"Yes. I was safe from the world, just not from him."

I struggled with the irony, then picked up my bat and walked down the hall to the last bedroom in the house. I turned the knob slowly and pushed open the door. In front of me, standing against the window, was a ghost image of my mother. Her stare was empty. On the floor in the room were coffee mugs half full of wine; I picked up the mugs and started smashing them against the wall.

"I hate this," I yelled. "I hate this."

Judith asked me what was happening, and before I could answer the brilliant, white light from outside the window disintegrated the wall and sucked out my mother. My body convulsed. My chest felt as though it had been torn open by a knife.

"She's dead!" I cried out to Judith. "The men killed my mom."

"Keep breathing," Judith said.

"She couldn't help me," I cried. "She wasn't strong enough... oh, God, it wasn't her fault... she wasn't strong enough. I'm sorry, Mom. I'm so sorry I blamed you."

"Keep breathing, Dawn. The shaking can't hurt you, but you have to keep breathing."

"My mom's dead. The light took her. Judith, I can't stand this pain. My chest feels like it's bleeding."

"Ask the light if it can help take the edge off."

My attention was drawn to the top corner of the room. Hovering there, like an angel of light, was the image of Anne.

I doubled over in tears. "Oh, God, she's always been here."

"Who?"

"Anne's here. She's always been here." I tried to catch my breath. "I've been so ashamed of my feelings for her, but this relationship kept me alive. It kept me alive."

Judith's voice was somber. "You don't have to be ashamed of your love for Anne. You don't ever have to be ashamed of that."

Judith loaded my hand with tissue. "What do you need to do next?"

I looked around. My mind was filled with light. The only dark left was the disintegrating structure of the house.

"What's happening, Dawn?" Judith asked.

"The house has been filled with light." I said. "It can't hurt me any more."

I calmed myself down and opened my eyes. I was shaking from head to toe, the grief from my mother's death still lingering.

"I'm still here," I said as I looked around her office. "I didn't lose my mind."

"No, you didn't lose your mind, and if you haven't lost your mind by now, you're never going to."

I was too weak to stand. "Judith, it feels like my mom just died. What if she's dead? What if the Christ light really just took her?"

"Your mother died when you were five. You're just finally strong enough to realize it."

"I don't know if I can get up," I said.

"You're fine," she said. "The worst is over and you survived it."

I knew I wasn't fine. But, I also knew what Judith was doing. She was showing me I was going to be all right by not reacting to my symptoms. I stood up still shaking, took a few deep breaths and hugged her good-bye.

I went home and walked into the kitchen.

"Judith let you leave like this?" Phil said. "You look like you've seen a ghost."

"I saw about five of them." I poured a glass of water and sat down at the table. My hands were still trembling and my chest was aquiver. I told Phil about the image and how the feelings were so present, I still feared my mom had died.

I went up to the nest and sat down at my desk, picked up the phone and dialed my mother's number. After three rings she picked up. When I heard her voice, I hung up the receiver. Tears of relief rolled down my face, followed by tears of longing. I needed a mother. I needed to be able to stay on that phone and tell my mom what had just happened, and I needed her to understand, hold me in her arms and tell me everything was going to be all right.

I looked at the phone and ran through the possibilities. For my mother to understand me, she would have to accept what had happened to me, and I knew in my heart that that just wasn't going to happen. I pushed away the phone and decided it was in my best interest not to call.

The next week marked the beginning of May and I felt as though my body chemistry was again changing. I could tolerate only fruits and vegetables. My thirst increased and I craved lemon water. I knew I was going through another type of cleansing—and it felt like the final rinse. I was about to discover the reason for my calling and the idea still made me nervous. I calmed myself by looking at Anne's picture. If God was as gentle as she was, I had nothing to fear.

I woke up one morning and pulled out her photo. My capacity to love her was still growing and I was realizing things about her that I hadn't realized before. Just a few months ago, I'd thought if she loved me, she would have stayed in contact. Now I was starting to believe that she didn't stay in contact because she loved me. Samantha walked in and jumped in my bed.

"What are you looking at?" she asked.

I showed her the picture of Anne holding a rabbit. "Do you see God in this picture?"

"Yeah," she said. "It's the rabbit."

I looked at the photo. The rabbit did look more present than Anne.

"Why do you look at her picture?" Samantha asked.

"I guess it reminds me of something I'm supposed to remember."

"What's that?"

"I don't know. When I remember it, I'll let you know."

She giggled and crawled under my arm as I pulled the blanket around her shoulders.

"Samantha, what do you think God is?"

"I thinks it's an invisible power," she said.

"Have you ever seen God, besides in rabbits?"

"I see God everywhere." I held her closer, giving her the security of a warm parent while I asked the questions of a frightened child.

"If God wanted to talk to you, would that scare you?" I said.

She giggled. "It would surprise me, but it wouldn't scare me."

"What do you think God would want to say?"

"I think God just wants people to feel better."

"And how does He do that?"

"He breaks open their love box and gives them a newer, cleaner one. So people can hold more love."

I stared at the ceiling, wondering what well of knowledge she so easily tapped.

"Does it hurt to have your love box opened?"

"No. It's the best thing that could ever happen to you."

That weekend it began to happen. It was Friday morning, the nineteenth of May, and Philip and Michael were leaving early for a weekend fishing trip. Michael came in and kissed me good-bye. I looked at the clock: 5:00 a.m. I rolled over and went back to sleep, and in my light slumber, I dreamed of pairs of large boa constrictors intertwined in a line blocking me as I tried to leave my home. There was a pair of snakes intertwined on my lawn, on my garage floor, and on the brick patio entrance to my house. The dreams weren't frightening, just unusual and vivid.

I awoke at 7:00 am and went in to take a shower. As the steam rose toward the ceiling, I began to notice my body felt lighter, and my head felt as though it was expanding. As the day went on, I continued to get the sensation of being lifted up, as if I was in a high-speed elevator being pulled away from gravity. At times it made me dizzy and I often had to lay down and rest, but I knew I wasn't sick and I dreaded what was coming. I left a message with Judith and tried to eat some lunch, but the food I ate went right through me and for the rest of the day all I could tolerate was juice and water.

Judith called that evening. I told her how I was feeling and described the dreams about the snakes. "Do you think the snakes represented an abuse memory?"

"No. I don't think you're in individual consciousness anymore. Snakes are a universal symbol of rebirth. And I'll have to check, but I believe snakes intertwined is the symbol of man's interconnection with the Divine. The dream may be a foreshadowing to the levels of consciousness you are entering."

"I don't like this, Judith."

"I'm here this weekend if you need me. But I think the best thing to do is center your self. Check in with Madame and Elisa and fasten your seat belt."

I fed the girls dinner and we crawled into bed. I fell asleep at nine o'clock and was awakened at 4:00 a.m, the morning of May 20th.

The inside of my head felt as though it was being dilated — spreading open like the walls of a cervix in final labor. I closed my eyes and Madame appeared.

Get ready to write.

I grabbed a notebook, and sat up in bed. In my mind, Madame stood on what appeared to be the floor of space. She was to the right and a few feet in front of a large, clear, black hole that came up from the floor. The hole had a pulse. And I could see moving, clear particles of energy coming up from its center. I realized the image represented God to me. In the physics material I had read, the center of all creation was described as a black hole in space. And in my mind, it was the only concept of God I had.

When I was ready to write, Madame moved to the side, and feeling like a pauper at the feet of the king, I began to take dictation. The information communicated to me through telepathic words that rose up from the image of the center of creation and into my mind as I wrote. The message began.

The evolution of your species has begun. The Dawn of a new consciousness is here. Don't be frightened. You will receive everything you need to make your transformation safely. Watch for the signs. I have sent other messengers. They will appear soon. They will lead you through different stages as your species evolves.

Sound your trumpets. A new beginning has arrived.

The discomfort in my head began to subside. I closed my notebook and lay back in bed, humbled to the very core of my being.

The rest of that Saturday was marked by the same sensations of being elevated. I couldn't eat much. I was dizzy at times and the fatigue continued. By the afternoon, I noticed Samantha had been caught up in the same sensations.

"I feel funny, Mom. Like something's happening to my head." She slept most of the day, and that night before we went to bed, she turned to me with the most radiant smile. "Mom," she said, "God just opened my love box."

We were in the same level of consciousness, but I wasn't having the same experience as she was. The sensation of losing control of my senses, my will, and my body had me strung as tight as a wire on a high-pitched guitar. A few hours later, I fell asleep. At 4:00 a.m., I awakened to the same experience I'd had the morning before: the information emerging from an image that looked like the center of creation, a clear, black hole in space.

This is a delicate time. You need to take care of each other. There are brothers and sisters amongst you who now embody my energy. Find them. They know of the Light and they will have no prejudices. Let the people who know, lead. Trust them. They are me.

It is very important to watch for the leaders because one is not real. He will have prejudices. Do not follow prejudice. It can only hurt you. Do not follow prejudice. It is not real, it is not me.

There are people in your churches and synagogues that embody the light— follow them.

Do not follow prejudice was heavily emphasized, as if the telepathic words became louder and even more authoritative when those sentences were being communicated.

I was then told to clarify who I was as the writer of this message. I didn't know myself until the information entered my mind and I wrote it down. In contrast to the other messages, although I still felt I was aligned with God, I could tell by the centered feeling in my body and the softer tone that the "I" in this message referred to me personally.

I am a messenger, not a healer. Others will come to help heal you. Do not follow me. I am not who you are looking for. I can only give direction. Go to your churches or synagogues for your healers.

All will transform. Allow your pain to transform you as I have done. The more we volunteer to do this, the less pain we will call upon ourselves.

The third Morning: May 22, 3:17 a.m.

I was awakened by the same sensation in my head, but this time there was an image: an apocalyptic scene that showed the death of many, many people — souls rising from earth by some kind of massive annihilation. The terror that came with this vision was more intense than any fear I had known. I left my room and curled up in a ball on the floor of the nest. I was reduced to a trembling animal. Safety in this world seemed impossible. An hour later, my terror subsided, and I was again summoned to write.

This is not necessary. Spare your brothers and sisters this pain by learning to love now. Transform your individual consciousness by choice. There is time to prepare. There is time to breed the strong, the healthy. There is time to stop the apocalypse. There is time for a gentle change.

Do not panic, my child, liberation is near and there is time to do it peacefully.

I put down my pen and, slowly closed the notebook, awe struck, as if I had seen a ghost. I kept the notebook in my desk and didn't open it again for several weeks. I was so profoundly struck by the divinity behind these messages that I couldn't speak for days.

Chapter 13

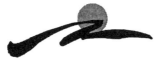

I didn't feel reborn. I felt like a fish that had been pulled from the pond and then tossed back in to relay a message from the pond keeper. There was no sensation of love or enlightenment. I still wasn't sure what the Light was, and my thoughts continued to be focused on when I would see my soul in Anne's.

"You sound like the Christian waiting for Jesus to return," Judith said in one of our sessions.

"Excuse me?" I didn't care much for the metaphor.

"You so passionately believe you will see Anne again that you're missing the point of her being gone."

"And what is the point?"

"The point is that she's not gone. Christ never left, so how can he come back? And Anne never left either. What you label Anne is really a part of you, but you're just not tuned into it, so you think she's not here."

I sat back in my chair. "On a thinking level, I understand that. I understand that what I saw in Anne was a part of me. What I yearn for every second I'm alone is me — the Christ light in me. But it still feels like what I want is Anne. And until that magical moment when I wake up and say 'Oh, I'm already her,' I will suffer."

"Are you still looking at her picture?"

"Yes, and I still can't tell you what I see in her, but I do know something is growing inside of me, and it feels like the love I have for her is who I am. And the stronger it becomes the more I know in my heart that I will see her again."

She nodded. "Dawn, I'll be honest with you. I don't know how much of your yearnings are childhood needs and how much of your yearnings are part of your transformational experience, but I don't think Anne has any reason or desire to return to Southern California."

"That might be the case, but this journey isn't over until I see her again."

"Then why don't you go out and find her. I'm sure with your resources you could track her down."

"I'm sure I could, and I've thought about it. But if I try to control this, all I'm going to find is disappointment."

"Probably."

"Anyway, what would I say to her? When she left, I just wanted to stay in contact with her. Now, I want to crawl in her bed and lie naked in her arms."

Judith's eyebrow shot up. "Excuse me for asking, but I didn't think this relationship was sexual for you."

"It's not. I don't want to have sex with her. I just want to lie naked in her arms."

She rubbed her forehead. "I'm still not clear."

"I'm tired and I'm lonely, and I want go back to the naked trust where I was safe and I was loved."

"And that was with Anne."

"Judith, I touched something when I was with her, something very loving and peaceful deep inside of me that I have never felt before. And I need to feel that again. I need to go home in her arms, back to that place so I can catch my breath and get the strength to go on with my life."

"Dawn, do you think Anne has those feelings for you?"

"Do I think Anne wants to lie naked in my arms?"

"Do you think Anne yearns to see you the way you yearn to see her?"

"That's my fantasy. But I don't think it's realistic."

"What do you think is realistic?"

"I don't know, but I don't think Anne's having the same experience. And I think she has found somebody to lie naked in her arms."

She set back her shoulders. "What makes you think that?"

"Lately, when I think of Anne, I get a vision of a man standing behind her. He's over her left shoulder. They look like they're together."

The energy between us shifted as if she was holding something back. "You know something don't you?"

She gave me a blank stare.

"Don't play that game with me. You've heard from her, haven't you?"

She paused. "I haven't heard from her, but I have heard of her."

"What?"

"We have a mutual friend in Oregon. She received a letter from Anne last week. Apparently, she's traveling with a man, and they are heading up to Canada for the summer. I don't know what kind of relationship they're in, but it sounded to me like they were just travel companions."

I ran my hands over my face. "Canada. How long is she going to be there?"

"I don't know, but I know she has no intention of returning here."

I couldn't tell which emotion was stronger, the relief of hearing something about her, or the disappointment that she was thousands of miles away and not returning here.

"Dawn, maybe the image is trying to tell you it's time to be with your man. I'm sure Philip would be happy to have you lie naked in his arms."

"It's not the same."

"I realize it's not the same, but I think it's time for you to start putting some of this energy into your marriage. You have three children at home, and the best thing for them is for you and Philip to stay together."

I didn't like what I was hearing, but it was the only thing left that made any sense. Judith was right. I could finish my process with the use of Anne's picture, and in the meantime try to find relief from my loneliness and put some energy back into my marriage.

Phil's birthday was at the end of June. Wanting to make the occasion romantic, I booked a room at a local resort. The day before his birthday, I packed for the night, digging through a lingerie drawer I hadn't opened in years. Nursing gowns, nylons, Christmas socks, negligees, here we go: a silk, white teddy that said *Take me, but take me slowly.* I put the teddy in my night bag and tossed in a pair of tall candles and his favorite perfume.

The sitter arrived in the afternoon, and we drove up to Newport Beach to a resort that overlooked the harbor. I told the hotel clerk it was a special occasion, and he upgraded our room to a suite.

We dropped off our night bags and walked out to the golf course to play nine holes. I wasn't very good at golf. It was a three-par course, and if I couldn't sink it in six, I knocked it in with my foot. Phil wasn't much better, but we were in our element, outside in the warm sun, having a good time.

The greens rolled over a hill above the harbor, and on the eighth hole we sat and watched the boats, dreaming of someday having our own. Phil wanted a small cabin cruiser to take the kids fishing in Catalina, while I day-dreamed of the nights in a berth with the windows open to a fresh sea breeze and the sounds of the water lapping against the hull.

The sun set behind Catalina Island, and we picked up our bags and played the last hole.

We dressed for dinner and went to our favorite restaurant, a fish house we used to frequent when we were first married. The maitre d' handed us the menu and took Phil's first order.

"I'll have a bucket of gin with a twist of lime," he said.

We both ordered swordfish. Mine came with water. His came with two more gins and a liter of wine. I was disgusted with him halfway through dinner, repulsed when the nightcap of cognac arrived.

I drove us back to the hotel grinding my teeth, not saying a word.

"What's wrong?" His voice was slurred.

I clutched the steering wheel. He sounded to me like my mother, and I had come too far in my process to still be living with my mother.

We walked into our hotel room. I zipped up my bag and tossed it in the closet. He lay down in the bed while I opened the amoire and checked the listing for a movie. *Legends of the Fall* sounded like an appropriate title. Phil passed out halfway through the video. I stayed up to watch a life more miserable than my own.

On the Fourth of July Phil caught his finger on a fence and had to cut off his wedding band. Then he ordered a keg of beer for the neighborhood party, and that was the last straw for me.

After breakfast, I got the kids situated upstairs and walked into the garage. Phil was working on his Fourth of July float: the Statue of Liberty on a wagon that Maxx was to pull.

"Can we talk?" I pulled up a stool.

"I don't know, can you talk?" He glared at me from his work bench.

"I want you to stop drinking."

He crossed his arms and spun around in his chair.

"Why?"

"Because I've lived with an alcoholic most of my life. And I choose not to live with one any more."

"I'm not an alcoholic."

"Then it shouldn't be difficult to stop drinking."

"I like to drink."

"Then it's time for you to decide what you like better, drinking or me."

His face turned red. "You're not exactly an attractive alternative to drinking."

"I'm sorry you feel that way, but you can either quit drinking, or I'll take the kids and leave."

"You're not taking those kids anywhere."

"Phil, with our gene pool, the last thing our children need is to be socialized around alcohol."

The muscles in his chest started to pulse. "And if I do decide to stop, what do I get?"

"What do you want?"

He kicked the bucket he was resting his foot on. "I want you to get out of your fuckin' head and start walking the face of this earth."

"I can do that."

"Can you? Because I don't want to spend another day with you sprawled out on the floor. I don't want to clean every fuckin' dish in this house because you're too apathetic to pick up after yourself, and I don't want to spent another night in our bed alone!"

"And if I agree, you'll stop drinking."

"For now. But my drinking isn't our problem, and if I have to eliminate it to prove that to you, I will."

"It's not all of the problem, but it's part of it, and we have to start somewhere."

He spun back towards his desk.

"And another thing," I said. "You might want to think about going to therapy. Because if you were healthy, you wouldn't have married me."

"That's for sure," he said.

We didn't speak for the rest of the day. I wasn't sure what his decision was until the next morning when I was sitting at the kitchen table reading the paper and the kids ran in from a trip with Phil to get donuts.

"Dad told us! Dad told us!" They said as they jumped in my lap.

"Dad told you what?"

They all started talking at once. I quieted the little ones and asked Samantha to explain.

"Dad said that it upsets you when he drinks beer, and that he didn't think his drinking was a very good example for us kids, so he decided to quit." Samantha started to cry. "I think that's the nicest thing."

Phil walked in and stood in the doorway. I looked up at him.

"It's the nicest thing anybody has ever done for me," I said.

I saw the Light twice that summer. The image was now an Angel of Light that stood a few feet from my body and was as large as I was.

Believe in her. The message it left was about Anne. I knew I couldn't give up. To see my soul in hers and finally reunite with that part of me, I knew I had to believe in her the way she believed in me — with the absolute faith that my truth would prevail.

Judith's skepticism and pragmatic advice was starting to feel more like another obstacle on my journey than help towards my destination. Our sessions were now spent in an escalating frustration, with me trying to convince her to have faith and believe, and her trying to communicate that she believed in me but not necessarily in Anne.

I came in for a session one afternoon, after taking the kids to the beach. I still had some sand on my feet that I didn't bother to fully brush off. I plopped down in her chair.

"I'm sick of coming here," I said. "I'm not at peace. I'm still afraid the Christ light is trying to invade me, and every time I try to believe in Anne I get distracted by doubts, theories and other people's voices."

"What is it that you're trying to believe in?"

"That I'll see her again. That she loves me as deeply as I love her. That emotionally she never left, she's a part of me and I'm not in this world alone." I set down my keys and leaned forward. "And when I hear her voice in my head, I can hear her telling me that it's all true. She tells me to believe, to have faith and to trust in what we shared."

"Then why don't you believe?"

"Because it's been two years since I've seen her and it's extremely unlikely that she's going to pop into my life, validate any of this, and then let me lie naked in her arms so I can go back to my soul. I'm deranged, Judith, and I'm getting worse."

"You're not deranged, but I think the voice you're hearing goes beyond Anne."

"I know it goes beyond Anne. But how can I believe in the voice if I can't believe in her?"

"How can you not believe in her?"

"Because I don't think you do." I stood up and paced. "Don't you see how hard it is to believe in this process when I can't see the conviction in your eyes? I need to believe in this with all my heart, and when I look at you every week, all I see are the variables."

"What variables do you see in me?"

"I don't think you like Anne. I think you think she flaked out on me. That she's selfish and ambivalent and that she doesn't have the capacity to love me as much as I love her. And I think that you half-heartedly believe in me. Part of you thinks this is my spiritual path and the other half of you believes it's a fantasy I created to try and get my childhood needs met."

She nodded.

"But, Judith, you didn't feel the love I felt with her. And I know that I shared it. That's why Anne didn't close our relationship. In her heart, she knew it wasn't over."

"It sounds like you do believe in her."

"I do until I look at you and start doubting myself. And I realize that's probably my own projection, but, Judith, this path didn't take me away from Anne, it took me back to her, and there must be a reason for that."

"I agree."

I sat down on the edge of my chair. "Then tell me that. I need to hear that you believe in me like she did. That you have faith that I'm doing the right thing."

"I do have faith in you. And I think you are doing the right thing. Your relationship with Anne is teaching you about your capacity to love and trust. The only place where I think we differ is that I don't think that ability should be contingent on Anne."

I clenched my teeth. "You keep saying that, but I don't know how I can trust with all my heart that it was real in me if I'm not sure it was real in her."

"How can it not be real? You experienced it."

"Yes, but I also believed it was real that my father would never hurt me. And he did."

"And so did Anne, but that doesn't mean that you didn't also experience love with both of them."

I turned away and stared out the window.

"Dawn, I experience Anne differently than you did, but I have found your descriptions of her to be accurate and well balanced. Anne was a very compassionate person, and she was also confused, afraid, and searching for something she couldn't find here. But I also believe that she loved you. That as much as you took her for your mother, she took you for a daughter. It would be easy to do."

"Then why am I so frustrated over all this?"

"I'm not sure. Close your eyes."

"I'm not in the mood."

"You're never in the mood."

"You sound like my husband." I thrust back in my chair and closed my eyes.

"Okay, go to the place where you believe. Where you hear Anne's voice and trust that she loved you. When you're grounded in that place, I want you to then go to the other, the place of doubt, and tell me what you feel."

"I feel fear."

"Okay, go back to the place where you hear Anne's voice. Then go back again to the place of doubt. I want you to do that several times and notice what you do to make the shift."

I went through the suggestion in my head and noticed the dropping point from faith was a question. I opened my eyes and looked at Judith.

"It's a question. When I start questioning myself, I drop into fear."

"Then stop questioning yourself."

"That doesn't sound very rational."

"Faith isn't rational. There's nothing logical about it. It's an intrinsic belief in the unknown and the unknowable, and that's why it's so difficult for people to have faith."

"But what if I'm believing in something that doesn't exist?"

"Then you're questioning yourself."

I nodded and smiled.

"Your assignment this week," she said, "is to stay in the place in your mind where you hear the voice of faith."

The voice of faith, that I could get to by imaging what Anne would say, now felt strong and clear, and rooted me in my own compassion. The sympathy I felt for myself over the abuse I endured in my childhood was now as sad as it had happened to one of my children. I cried often. I cried because I was an innocent child raped by my father, and I wept for the insanity of a group of grown men molesting me as a child. I cried over Anne and how difficult therapy had been, and sometimes I turned over in bed and cried for no reason in the safety of Philip's arms. He was sober every night and I'd never known such consistency.

In September, the kids went back to school and my body made another shift. The Kundalini energy began to rise, welling up from the center of my body like large gas bubbles. For weeks I felt as though it was expanding my chest. My heart warmed with the sensation of heat, then a quickening of ecstasy.

In October the energy rose to my throat. There was a constant tightness around my larynx, and at times it was difficult to swallow. The nights were becoming uncomfortable and the unusual sensations were making me nervous. The more I resisted them the worse they became, so I tried to slow the energy down by stopping the Twelve Hands of Tao Mo and relaxing with a massage. I called Jill at the Ritz Carlton and booked an appointment for a massage.

"What brings you here in October?" Jill said, "It's not your birthday."

I lay down on the table, and she covered me with a sheet. "Have you heard of the Kundalini energy?"

"Yes."

"It's rising in my body and it's driving me crazy."

She laughed. "You know, most of the people I know would love to be having the spiritual experiences you're having."

"I don't love it."

"Are you resisting the energy?" she asked.

"Well, I'd like to be able to control it."

"Try to ride with it, instead of against it. How's your breathing?"

"It's sporadic. Sometimes I feel like I need to catch my breath."

"Sometimes energy shifts will calm down if you start breathing into your stomach instead of your chest."

I remembered being told the same thing by Russ.

"Have you ever heard of a place called Esalen?" she said.

"Isn't it a spiritual retreat up in Big Sur?"

"Well, kind of. They have human development workshops. I think I've seen a couple classes on transformation and energy shifts. It might be helpful for you to check it out."

"Have you been there?" I asked.

"I go as often as I can. It makes me feel whole again."

She moved down my spine to the small of my back. "I have a fall schedule of workshops," she said. "I'll give it to you before you leave."

The energy in my head increased over the next two weeks as I felt depressed, then angry; elated, then enlightened. There were moments when the world seemed clear and I was me, not my past. My hearing became hypersensitive and my eyes felt constantly dry.

The energy welled like a pool at the crown of my head, and on the first of November, I felt a warm stream of energy flow out the top of my skull. My seventh chakra had opened. I now felt like an open channel in a river much larger than myself.

That night I opened my journal and wrote about the sensations; at the end of the first paragraph a sentence popped out:

Go to where Anne is.

I didn't know where Anne was, so I wrote down several question marks, assuming the sentence had come from my imagination.

Two days later, I awoke to a message:

Go to the big trees.

I didn't pay much attention until I received the same message again the following day.

Go to the big trees.

I thought the message had something to do with the energy shifts. That I needed to spend some time around big trees to help ground the new energy.

I didn't act on it until the third day.

Go to the big trees.

The big trees meant Big Sur to me. That was where the groves of redwoods met the mid-coast of California. But the biggest redwoods in California were in the Sequoia National Park, so I told Phil about the messages and asked if he wanted to take the kids and go to the sequoia forest.

"Sure, as long as Maxx can go," he said.

The kids were out of school the following Thursday and Friday, so we penciled in a four- day vacation and I called and rented a motor home.

I played phone tag with Judith, trying to reschedule my next appointment. On Saturday afternoon, she got in touch with me. We changed our appointment from Tuesday to Wednesday and before I hung up, I told her about the messages.

"Judith, I keep getting this message to go to the big trees."

"Go to Big Sur," she said.

"Why?"

"Anne's there."

My heart started to race. "How do you know?"

"Last week I was talking to my friend up in Oregon. Anne stopped there on her way down from Canada. She was heading for a place called Esalen, a retreat in Big Sur where workshops are held."

I sat down. "You're kidding."

"No, apparently she's going for a month. I was surprised because I thought their workshop only lasted a week, but my friend Carolyn said the workshop she was taking lasted, I think, until the middle of December." There was a long pause. "Are you still there?"

"Yes. This is so strange."

I told Judith I'd see her on Wednesday, hung up the phone and ran upstairs to my desk. On the top of the pile was the Esalen fall schedule Jill had given me after my massage with her last week. I looked through the catalog for a workshop that lasted a month and found only one for the fall season, a certified program for massage therapy that was scheduled to begin Sunday, November 14th. Good, I had over a month to figure out what I needed to do.

I went downstairs and told Phil what had happened.

"Great. I'll take you there," he said.

"What?"

"Instead of going to the sequoias next weekend, we'll take the motor home up the coast. We can drop you off at Esalen on Sunday, and I'll drive back with the kids."

"You'd do that?"

"Sure, I'll take you wherever you want to go."

It was my answer. If there was a workshop open, I'd go next week. I walked back upstairs and called Esalen; they had one workshop still open, a week course on intimacy that began the evening of the fourteenth. I booked the workshop and gave them my credit card number. It was all happening so fast, each step feeling so right, I never once questioned what I was doing.

I called Jill that night and told her what had happened.

"If you're lucky," she said, "you'll be put in the Big House. It's right on the cliff looking over the ocean, and if you stay there, you'll probably only have one roommate. You might want to call and request it."

I didn't feel the need to call; at that point I was living on faith. "Do I need to bring a sleeping bag?"

"No, the rooms have bedding and towels, but they don't have phones. Tell your husband if he wants to reach you he has to call the office and they leave a message on the message board."

I thanked her, hung up and went down to make dinner.

My fear didn't set in until I crawled into bed. Would she really be at Esalen, and if she was, what would it be like to see her again? Would I love her as much in person as I had in my mind, and would she love me as much as I thought she did when she left?

I prayed hard that night. I prayed that somehow she knew I was coming. That she could receive some warning so my reunion with her would be the happy occasion I needed it to be.

I awoke at 6:00 a.m., my chest bubbling with an urgency to write. I picked up my journal and the message spewed out, as it had in the past — a stream of automatic writing.

She knows you're coming. She's ready to heal her heart. Spend time with her. You will heal her as she heals you. Let the light work through you. Let the light in and give it to Anne. You are meant to heal her as she heals you. Remember, you were meant and sent to heal her.

I shook my head as I took down the message. Could this path get any stranger? I closed my journal and lay back in bed, feeling humbled by the message, not worthy to accomplish the mission.

Philip woke up and I crawled under his arm; his touch was softer now, his advances less aggressive. I moved up on his chest to kiss him, then the kids broke through the door and jumped in our bed.

"We're starved. Can we have some pancakes?"

Phil moaned while I jumped out of bed and raced the kids to the kitchen.

On Tuesday, I went to my session with Judith. She didn't look good and neither did I. I sat down in my chair, my legs bouncing up and down on the floor as I told her about the month-long massage class I thought Anne might be taking and the workshop on intimacy I'd reserved for myself.

Her face turned pale as she shook her head. "I don't know. That doesn't sound right. Carolyn never said anything about Anne being interested in body work. And maybe my dates were wrong. I don't know. Was it going to be this soon? "

"Judith, you sounded so clear on the phone."

"I just don't remember if the workshop was a month or two months. I think it was two months... but I don't know."

Her confusion appeared layered; there was too much energy behind it for this to just be about Anne's plans.

"What is going on with you? Are you concerned about me going up there?"

"No, that's not it. When we got off the phone, I questioned whether I should have told you. But this is such an unusual case. Most therapists don't leave their practice. And when they do, they have an address or phone number where they can be reached. I've tried other ways to help you close this relationship with Anne, but nothing else has worked. I know you need to see her for your process with her to be over."

"Then what's the problem?"

She gave me a tearful look. "I don't know, give me a second to check this out." She stared past me and went inward, her eyes continuing to fill until a tear ran down her cheek.

"I guess it's the idea of your process being over. I know the whole reason I'm a therapist is so people can come in here, get better and then leave, but when you've spent time with people you enjoy, it's difficult to see them go. I want you to be able to complete your process, but there is also a part of me that hopes Anne isn't there so we can go on."

I started to cry. When the baby is delivered, you have to say goodbye to your obstetrician, and Judith had supported me through so much it seemed almost unfair that she wouldn't be with me to share the last leg of my journey. She handed me a tissue.

"There have been too many losses," I said.

"It's part of the process, Dawn."

She handed me another tissue and sat back in her chair.

"What's the best and worst thing that can happen to you at Esalen?" she asked.

The change of subject calmed me. "The best thing would be that I'm healed, Anne's healed and the relationship is healed. And I guess the worst thing is that she somehow rejects me."

"She already has rejected you. She left, and you grew up on your own. You have yourself as an adult now, and what happened before can't happen again."

"It feels like it can."

"That's your five-year-old talking, and she had no business going up to Esalen to meet Anne. This is for you as an adult."

I sat up in my chair. "I can't take the five-year-old?"

"No, you can't. Dawn, that child needed the relationship with Anne in order to get your attention. She needed to love and trust somebody enough so that you could love and trust yourself. But she has you now. She doesn't need Anne and she doesn't need you to abandon her for Anne. Leave her at home."

"All right."

"How are you going to make sure she's not there?"

"I'll check in with myself often and imagine her home with my kids."

"Good, because if you end up on the floor at Esalen, you'll have to call Karen. I'm not going to drive up to Big Sur, pick you up, and take you to the hospital. I'm going to tell you to send the five-year-old home and handle this like an adult."

I smiled at her. Her tough love never felt so good.

"Dawn, I want you to hear this. You are an adult. You can be hurt or disappointed, but nothing Anne says or does can devastate you. Leave the child at home—she doesn't belong there."

I came home and started to pack. The kids and I were going through their clothes, and Phil was downstairs with a gentleman from a recruiting company. He was signing the final contract with an executive search firm—another sign that our lives were finally getting back to normal.

"I'm going to walk Mr. Evan to his car and then take Maxx for a walk," he yelled from downstairs.

"Okay," I said as I counted out the twelve pairs of underwear Erica had packed for our four-day vacation. I went into her drawer and tried to balance her wardrobe. I was ready to start on Michael's clothes when the phone rang, and I ran into my bedroom to answer it. All I could hear was sobbing.

"He's dead...he's dead!" Phil wailed from the car phone.

I scanned my mind for the kids. They were home. They were safe.

"What happened?"

"Maxx was just hit by a car. It hit him hard. Oh, God, he's dead. I know he's dead."

"Where are you?"

"I'm in the car, I'm taking him to the vet, but Maxx isn't moving. He's dead! He's dead!" He sounded like an eight-year-old who had just lost his father.

"He's going to be okay Phil. Maxx is going to be okay. Take a couple of deep breaths and tell me where you're going."

"His tail moved! Maxx wagged his tail. He wagged his tail!"

"He's telling you he's going to be all right. Maxx is going to be all right. Now where are you going, so I can meet you there?"

"No. No. I want you to stay with the kids, and please don't tell them what happened. Please don't tell them." Samantha was standing next to me listening to the conversation.

"Are you sure you don't want me to meet you?"

"Yes, I'm sure. I'll call you when I get there."

Michael and Erica walked into the room. "What's happening?" Michael said.

"Maxx was just hit by a car," Samantha said.

Erica and Michael broke into tears. I walked over and held them.

"Maxx is going to be fine. Dad took him to the hospital and the doctors are taking good care of him."

We spent the next hour huddled on the couch distracting ourselves by watching sitcoms. The phone rang and we all ran to answer it. I picked it up.

"Maxx is alive," Phil said. "There's no broken bones, but he's having some trouble breathing from the shock. The doctors want to keep him overnight, and if he's okay tomorrow, we can take him home in the afternoon."

"He'll be okay, Phil. I know he will."

"I think so, too, but it doesn't look like we'll be able to make the trip."

"That's fine. I'll cancel the motor home, and if Maxx is okay, I'll drive up on my own on Sunday."

That night was sleepless. Phil called every hour to check on Maxx, and every time he closed his eyes, he saw him being hit by the car. "Maxx ran right into that car," he kept saying. "He ran right into it." He tossed and turned. "I should have had him on a leash. Why didn't I have him on a leash?"

I fell asleep just before dawn, and when I awoke, Phil was gone. He called after breakfast to say that Maxx was standing up. His breathing was still labored, but he could walk.

"I slept in his kennel with him," Phil said. "I chewed on his ear to make sure he knew who I was."

"Maxx knows who you are, honey."

"I'm going to stay out here for awhile."

"Okay, I'm going to cancel the motor home and see if we can get back our deposit."

"Dawn, I still want you to go to Esalen."

"We'll see."

Phil came home for lunch and went straight to bed. I had put away the kids' clothes and was heading down to clean the kitchen when the phone rang. I picked up before it woke Phil.

"Hello." ·

"Mrs. Kohler?"

"Yes."

"This is Doctor Klein, the veterinarian. Maxx is having some real trouble breathing and I'd like to send him to another facility where they can put in a chest tube until we can assess the lung damage."

Phil picked up the other phone halfway through the conversation. "I'll be right there," he said. He ran out of the house without saying goodbye.

"Is Maxx going to be okay?" Michael said.

"Yeah, Maxx will be okay. Whatever happens, Maxx will be okay."

I finished cleaning the kitchen, and we went to buy groceries. The kids were in good spirits as they ran down the aisles. My pace was slower, my chest filled with trepidation. I bought them the ice cream sandwiches I usually denied and, sensing my weakness, they pushed for some gum. My bill was twenty dollars more than it normally was, but my kids were happy and relatively quiet.

We had loaded the groceries and were headed back home when Phil's van pulled up next to me at the light. His shoulders were shaking, and he was hunched over the steering wheel. He looked over at me and mouthed the words.

"He didn't make it," he said. "He didn't make it."

I looked at him and moaned. I would have given up my chance of ever seeing Anne again if God would have just brought back his dog.

Chapter 14

After Maxx died, I didn't know what to expect. I wasn't sure if Anne would be at Esalen. Or if I could physically stand another loss. But I went anyway — because I had to, and because Phil insisted.

I loaded the refrigerator with casseroles and desserts, trying to anticipate my family's needs while I was gone, trying to feel less guilty about leaving. After breakfast on Sunday, I said goodbye to the kids and checked in with my inner five-year-old. I imagined her on the couch eating popsicles with Michael and asked her to stay with him and not creep into my consciousness while I was gone. For the next week, I would need to be an adult.

Phil walked me out to the dog van. It still smelled like Maxx.

"Are you sure you're going to be okay?" I said.

"I'll be fine. The kids are a good distraction."

I leaned over and kissed him. "I'm coming back, you know."

He smiled. "I know."

Melissa Etheridge sang me up the coast, her voice drowning out any thoughts of my own. When I hit the center of the state, I turned off the music and focused my attention on the change in scenery. The ocean below the rocky cliffs was calm, hugging the coast like a big blue safety pad as my van tilted around the curves of the winding coast highway. I swerved into fog banks and then back into sunshine, the extremes feeling much like my senses.

The redwoods were now lining the highway, and the fog dissipated as I came out around a narrow bend and saw the small wooden sign:

Welcome to Esalen
by Reservation Only

My heart started to race. What was I in for? A middle-aged man with his hair tucked behinds his ears directed me to the registry and told me where to park.

I stepped out of the van and looked around. A brilliant green lawn sprawled through the grounds, each blade of grass calling notice to its life. I walked past some pine trees and out to the cliff. Below me was the majestic Big Sur coast line: steep curves of jagged rock embraced by the pliable blue waters that foamed white at its borders. A lone bird glided down a wind current; from below came the bark of an otter.

I walked through the vegetable garden and over to the office feeling nervous yet, strangely at peace. Everything in nature told me she was there. Everything around me seemed part of who I was.

I walked to the counter and gave the clerk my name. I thought of asking about Anne, but then my attention was drawn to the computer behind the clerk. Taped to the monitor was a handwritten note: *TRUST* I heeded the message.

The clerk handed me my keys. "You're in the Big House," he said. "Here's a map to your room and the schedule for your workshop."

Back past the garden and over a walking bridge that was dampened by the mist of a nearby waterfall, I picked up a path to the Big House, a large, country-style home that stood on the cliff. A red brick patio surrounded the house and redwoods with roots that curved above the ground extended high above the arch of the two-story building. My room was upstairs, a small bedroom at the beginning of the hall with an old, wooden desk against one wall and two twin beds pushed up against two windows that looked out over the ocean. I put down my luggage and opened the windows; the sounds of the ocean poured in with the fresh air.

There was no sign of a roommate, so I put away my stuff and walked to the cafeteria to get something to eat. On the way, I checked the message board, a piece of framed cork that hung outside the office. There was nothing with Anne's name on it, but there was a message for me. I pulled it down and opened it. The message was from Jill, the masseuse at the Ritz Carlton who during my last massage, told me about Esalen, and gave me the fall schedule.

> *No one can fail who seeks to reach the truth.*
> *-A Course in Miracles-*
> *Love,*
> *Jill*

Warmed by her kindness, I put the note in my pocket and went in for dinner.

The cafeteria was a rustic lodge with benches lining a window that overlooked the pool. In the rear of the room was a lounge area, a raised platform with sitting pillows sprawled around wooden coffee tables. I went through the buffet line and sat by the window. There was no sign of Anne.

I ate three bites of stew, pushed away my plate and pulled out the schedule for my workshop. The first session was to begin at eight that night, and would meet for two hours every morning, afternoon and evening. Wednesday was the only night I had free.

I looked at my watch: a quarter to seven. Outside the kitchen was a pile of dirty dishes; I added my plate and walked outside. The air was brisk and still, the night too dark to see. I turned on my flashlight and walked back to my room. A duffel bag was on the other bed and a light jacket hung in the closet.

At eight o'clock, I went downstairs to the unfurnished living room where my group was scheduled to meet. The workshop leaders greeted us warmly at the door: Terry, a handsome man in his early forties wearing jeans and a button down shirt, and Gina, a gray-haired, full-bodied woman wearing a sea-green, long sweater and flowing, long shirt. They both had psychotherapy practices in Massachusetts and came to Esalen twice a year to lead workshops.

Inside the door were stacks of pillows; each person grabbed one as they entered and set them down in a large circle on the carpet. I sat next to a man who looked like Jay Leno. He smiled warmly as he firmly shook my hand.

"Hi, I'm Paul."

I introduced myself and we greeted the people around us. So far, there were about twenty of us, men and woman from all over the world.

Terry and Gina gave a brief introduction of the intimacy workshop, then asked each of us to share why we had decided to take the course. I wasn't about to tell them I'd picked it on a whim so I'd have something to do while I looked for my therapist. The floor opened to Paul.

"I was supposed to come here with my wife," he said, "but she couldn't make it. We've been married for fifteen years and would like to find ways to have a more intimate relationship." He finished and turned to me.

"I've been dealing with childhood sexual abuse," I said. "And I'd like to get out of my childhood." The group nodded compassionately and we moved to the next person.

When group was over, I went up to my room. My roommate, who was taking the same workshop, came into the room behind me. She introduced herself as Catherine, a bubbly, middle-aged therapist with long, curling, red hair, who worked with troubled teenagers in a high school in Massachusetts.

We hit it off right away. By midnight, we were as comfortable as sisters.

In the morning, Catherine and I met Paul in the lobby and the three of us went up for breakfast. I hadn't slept much. Every step toward the cafeteria was making me more nervous. We stopped at the message board so I could put up a note for Anne. I wanted to warn her I was there, give her some time before she saw me.

I was full after a few bites and my heart fluttered every time the door opened. If Anne was there she would have to come here to eat, and in two meals I hadn't seen her. By the end of breakfast, I had a headache. To hell with trust. I needed the facts.

I excused myself from the table and walked into the office.

"Excuse me," I said to the clerk. "I think a friend of mine is here. Could you check for her on the roster?"

"Sure, what's her name?"

"Anne Myers."

"That name sounds familiar." He grabbed a clipboard and scanned through the workshops.

"No... No, I don't see her. But I recognize the name. I think she left yesterday."

The lump in my throat dropped into my stomach. I'd missed her by one day.

"I'm sorry. Is there something else I can do for you?" he said.

"No." I put on my sunglasses, walked out the door and tore my note to her off the message board. One day. How could I have missed her by one day?

I walked down to a rock on the lawn. Everything around me was still telling me she was there. *Shut up!* I screamed to the voice in my head. Give it up already. Maxx is dead and Anne's not here.

I walked over the bridge, past the house, down a flight of stairs onto a rocky beach.

I threw off my jacket and picked up some stones.

"Damn it! I don't deserve this shit anymore!" I burst into tears as I smashed the rocks into the water. "Why did Maxx have to die? And why did you bring me here?" I yelled to the sky. "Why?"

My tears turned to sobs as I sat on the rocks. "I don't want to be hurt anymore. Please. Please, let this be over."

The tears were still pouring down my face when I walked up to group. As we sat down in our circle, twenty-four pairs of eyes seemed to be staring at me. Terry addressed me as soon as the circle began.

"Dawn, this is a sacred circle, and it's safe if you want to share what's happening." I was so present in my emotions I couldn't control them.

"I saw this therapist," I cried, "whom I loved very deeply. She was helping me through my depression, but about six months after I remembered the sexual abuse, she quit her practice and left the country." There was gasp in the room. "We were very close and we never had closure. Last week, I heard she was here and the only reason I came up to take this class was so I could find her." My voice cracked as the woman next to me reached for my hand. "I asked for her at the desk this morning and they said I had missed her by one day."

The group winced.

"I'm sorry, Dawn." Terry, the workshop leader said. "I'm really very sorry."

I took a breath and composed myself. Gina, the other workshop leader addressed me warmly. "Dawn," she said, "The exercise this morning is to talk about the strength that enabled us to survive our childhood. Would you like to start?"

I wiped my eyes. "Hope. Hope enabled me to survive my child-hood. The hope that someday there would be an answer. That the world would somehow, someday, make sense. But I'm giving up on hope. Faith is driving me crazy, and I don't want to hear it in my head anymore."

A sigh of sadness echoed in the room. I looked at Paul to take the attention off of myself, and he picked up the question and it went around the circle. I listened to stories of people who survived on good behavior, on rebellion, and as caretakers to their parents. There where people who survived by running away and people who survived by submission. Each voice spoke a part of my truth. I had been all of them, just as they had been me.

When our morning session was over, we walked up for lunch. The anticipation of seeing Anne was finally over and the relief brought back my appetite. I loaded up a plate and went outside to eat with Catherine. It was a clear, warm day and the dry air made me thirsty. I set down my plate, downed a glass of water and went back to the cafeteria for another cup. While I was filling my glass from the spigot, a woman who resembled Anne walked by. Her tennis shoes and leggings were worn, the sleeves on her green sweat shirt were pushed up to her elbows. I stared at her back as she walked toward a table, holding my breath squinting for recognition. Was it Anne? Was my two-year nightmare about to be over? She crossed the room slowly, appearing taller than I remembered Anne, her gait more confidant. The woman's long, brown hair covered her face as she put down her plate. Then she turned to sit and pushed her hair behind her shoulders. I saw her face clearly. It was Anne. A smile returned to my face that I hadn't felt in years.

My mind went blank as I walked up to her chair.

"Hi," I said as I stood in front of her.

She looked up at me and slowly nodded. "I always knew I was going to see you again."

I just stared at her. Everything I needed to know I knew in that instant. Anne loved me, but not the way I had loved her.

She took a bite of her salad. "Sit down," she said, gesturing to the empty seat beside her.

I dropped down in the chair, my hands trembling. "I can't believe I'm seeing you. They told me at the desk you weren't here."

"I got here yesterday. But I'm in a residence program. They probably checked the workshops." She took another bite.

"What's the residency program?"

"It's a therapy program, and it's accredited by the state so I can use it for further training as a therapist. We work in the different maintenance departments during the day and we go to therapy groups at night. I think I'm in the laundry this week."

My stomach started to quiver, and she reached for my hand.

"It's okay. I knew I was going to see you again. And I just had to trust that when it was right the universe would somehow bring us back together."

"How do you two know each other?" said the man to her left.

"Dawn, this is Uray. He's a friend of mine."

"Hi, Uray." I looked back at Anne. I told her about the message to go to the big trees and the sequence of events that had brought me to Esalen.

She listened, cautiously amused. Still eating her plate of salad that sat on the rustic, dark, wooden table. The window behind her looked out over the brilliant green lawn and out to a calm, blue ocean. "Well, I'm working here," she said, "I'm not sure how much time we will have to spend together, but you're welcome to come eat with us, and on Wednesday night I don't have a session. We can get together then."

"That's good. I don't have a workshop on Wednesday night either." My body was still shaking. "I think I need some time to let this sink in," I said.

She nodded and I stood up and hugged her.

"It's good to see you," I said.

Her eyes began to warm. "It's good to see you, too."

"It was nice to meet you," I said to Uray. It was the first time we made eye contact. He was tall and blonde with a boy's pale, soft skin face in a man's broad-shoulder body.

"Nice to meet you," he said with an accent I couldn't distinguish.

I walked back to the Big House laughing at myself — at how my lack of trust brought on so much of my own suffering. I saw Catherine on the path that went through the garden and as we walked back to our room I told her about Anne.

"Was it strange? Was it awkward? Was she glad to see you?"

"Yes."

"Are you going to see her again?"

"Wednesday night we're going to meet. But I'll probably see her before then." I took off my jacket and picked up a towel. "Do you want to go to the hot springs with me?" I said.

"I'd love to, but I have some things I need to read."

I walked back over the bridge and past the garden. In front of the cafeteria I ran into Anne. Uray was a few feet away.

"Hi," I said. "I'm going to the hot springs. Do you want to come?"

She hesitated. "Well, I just found out I have the afternoon off, but I told Uray I would help him clean some rooms."

"Are you sure? I have a lot to tell you."

She looked back at him. "I don't know," she said. There was a long pause. "Okay, I'll meet you down there."

I waited for Anne at the front of the bathhouse, in awe that I was finally seeing her, relieved that I would have the chance to share with her all the things that had happened.

She walked up a few minutes later, and we went down to the baths, large tubs made of smooth, gray stones that stood on a deck that was perched out from the jagged cliffs, high above the coastline. The hot springs were bathing suit optional — and no one I saw opted for a suit. We took off our clothes and stepped in the tub. The sun was nearing the horizon, the ocean as calm as a morning sea.

Anne sat next to me. "This is a pretty good place for God to bring us back together," she said.

"Divine perfection,"

I gushed on about the path I had been on, telling her about the eulogy, the dream where I fell into her arms, and the message to love her with all my heart, soul, and mind. None of it seemed to be connecting, so I took a deep breath, calmed myself down and looked at her as my mind went still. She smiled at me as if she was enjoying the silence, and suddenly, a light reflected off the water and up into her face. For a moment, I was blinded by the glare, and when my vision cleared — I saw her soul. Her body appeared translucent and sitting adjacent to me was her soft, wise, compassionate soul, softly glowing at me as if I had entered another realm. The sight brought words to my mouth that were given to me.

"You were faith and spirit to me," I said, "and everybody kept telling me I wasn't going to see you again, but now that I have I am never going to lose you again."

"Who told you, you weren't going to see me again?"

I told her about Susan, the woman who did spiritual reading, and Karen, the therapist Anne had referred me to when she left. "Karen said your last letter to me was closure."

She shook her head. "No, no, it wasn't closure. And when I got your letter, I really wanted to write you back. I knew you thought I was just another person in your life who screwed you over, but every time I talked to my friends about it, they just kept telling me I had to let it go." She shook her head. "But it never felt right. I knew there was something about our relationship that just didn't translate into words, but if you hear something enough times you start to realize there's probably a reason for it."

I asked her if she had read the *Tibetan Book of the Living and Dying*. She hadn't, so I told her about the Tibetan practice of placing a teacher with a student until the student saw his or her soul in the teacher. And how I had used her picture to try and connect to that part of myself.

She leaned back against the tub. "I gave you a picture?"

"Yes, you did."

"What picture did I give you?"

"You were holding a rabbit."

"I was...?"

I splashed some water over my face. How could she have forgotten about the picture? I checked in with my body to see how I felt. My chest was heavy and hurting. The reality that she meant a lot more to me than I did to her was setting in. I started telling her about some of the other messages I'd received, but when I could see I was still not connecting, I cut myself short.

"I guess I'm just having an unusual life," I said.

"You really are."

"Anyway, enough about me. Are you all right?"

"Yeah, I really am. I've had a lot of fun the past two years. I came back from Australia, bought a van, and camped all through the West. It's been great."

"Did you come here with Uray?"

"Yes, but he's just a friend. I met a man from Germany about a year ago. We traveled through Canada together. And then were scheduled to come here, but his visa ran out and they wouldn't let him cross the border back into the States." She took a deep breath. "It's really hard to be here without him."

"What's his name?"

"Otto."

I nodded. "Next lifetime, I'm taking your path. It sounds a lot more fun than the one I've been on."

"Oh, it hasn't been all fun. It's really hard living with somebody in a van, and there are some issues with Otto that I came here to work on." She turned on a blast of cool water, then moved closer to me.

"How's therapy going?" she asked.

"Good. I've spent a lot of time working on my transferences with you. And I was told you probably had a few with me."

"They told you that, did they?"

I smiled at her. "Yes, they did."

"It's true. I had some issues that came out in our relationship that were part of my own process."

"What were your transferences?" I asked.

The energy changed. She was letting down and becoming more comfortable with me. "You were absolutely a daughter to me. And I knew what my leaving was going to put you through. Believe me, I know how much this hurt you." Her eyes filled with tears. I stepped over and held her and she welcomed the embrace.

"I received a message," I said. "A few days before I came here. It said you were ready to heal your heart."

"Oh, yes," she cried, "yes...yes. I have worried and wondered about you for a very long time."

Another wave of tears came up from her chest. I held her tightly, my senses not fully present, I was naked in her arms and the realization was overwhelming.

"It's okay," I said. "It's okay."

She pulled away. "I know it is."

I sat back and went inward. I was happy for Anne, but the reconnection I had longed for wasn't healing me. I was still alone. And she wasn't my answer.

A group of people joined us in the tub. We got out and walked to a vacant one.

I moved slowly, picked up my towel. There was too much to process, and I wanted to leave.

"I'm feeling kind of stuck," I said. "Maybe I should go back to my group."

She sat down in another tub. "Or you could stay here and just be stuck."

I accepted her invitation and climbed in the tub. I had come all this way. I might as well tell her how I felt.

"I know we had different experiences of each other," I said, "but part of mine was that I fell in love with you, and I fell into it deep."

"You really did, didn't you?"

"Yes, I did, and I know that was my own experience."

She nodded. "Isn't that all life is? Our own experience of it?"

I wished I hadn't stayed.

"I guess, but it's lonely to think I was in it alone."

"You weren't in it alone. And I don't think the love I experienced with you was any more or less. It was just different."

"How's that?"

"I knew from the first days we worked together that I had always loved you. I don't know in what past life or what relationship, and I don't need to know. But I have always loved you and always will."

Her words didn't register. I was still recovering from her not remembering she gave me her picture.

"What's going on with you and Philip? " she asked.

"Phil's a good man. I just thought that if I could somehow get my heart open through my relationship with you, I'd be able to love him more. I don't know if that makes sense anymore. But I used to think it did."

"So, what do you need from me?"

"I need to free myself. To let go of my fears in your arms so I know who I am."

She smiled. "I think we might be able to arrange that this week." She pointed to the sun as it touched the horizon, yellow and orange glowing from its borders. We waded to the edge of the tub and she put her arm around me. "It's beautiful, isn't it?"

"Yes, it is."

I let go of my thoughts and reached for her hand, weaving my fingers inside of hers, feeling how safe I was in her arms. Then I closed my eyes, aware of the sun setting in front of me, more aware of the one arising within me, the love for her that was filling my body like warm liquid pouring into an empty glass. It felt as though the love was overflowing, pouring out of the top of my head. The isolation I had been in for so long finally broke, the cells in my body awoke, and I took a breath of air that was lighter and fresher than I thought air could be.

"I'm glad you came," she said. "You have given me a very healing gift."

I nodded, moving my hand slightly, just enough to feel the skin on her fingers, just enough to feel the skin on my own.

The sun disappeared. "It still feels like there's something else I'm supposed to give you," I said.

"I don't know what that could be. You've already given me plenty."

We stayed together until the sky lost its glow, and by the time we left there was so much love in my body I could feel it beaming out my eyes and radiating from my skin.

I walked back to the Big House and caught the last minutes of my workshop. The word had spread that I'd found Anne, and when I entered the living room I was greeted with cheers.

"You look like a lit candle," said a woman from Missouri.

Paul came up and hugged me. "You're beautiful."

"Thank you." I was at peace.

We broke for dinner and then came back for our evening session, all of us grabbing our pillows and setting up our sacred circle.

The exercise of the evening was to go to the person you felt most uncomfortable with. The room scrambled for partners. Debbie, the woman who had sat next to me the night before, and I were left together by default. We both wanted the same guy, but Catherine got to him first, so we made good use of the time and talked about why he annoyed us.

I went to bed that night elated, woke up afraid. I had been wide open with Anne, exposed the way a small island is to the elements that surround it. Our relationship, now more than ever, was too intense to be causal. Until I could ground myself, I decided to avoid her. I went to the cafeteria early, ate fast, then took a walk with Catherine.

We came back for the morning group, and Gina ran the session, teaching us a physical exercise of positioning designed to help us be aware of whether we preferred to dominate or submit. Domination felt too aggressive. Submission was frightening.

Before lunch, I grabbed a towel from the laundry. I knew Anne worked there. Her work program included doing the laundry and cleaning rooms, and my heart was pounding as I walked up to the small building. I reached the door and, from the corner of my eye, saw Anne duck into the back. Oh shit—she was avoiding me. My heart began to race as if trying to run away from me; the despair opening in my chest was threatening to swallow me whole. I went to the bridge to regroup. This wasn't happening. This couldn't be happening. It was just my imagination—I needed to try again.

When I came back to the laundry room, she was folding some towels. I walked up and stood beside her, trying to say something clever, but nothing clever came out. Her attempts at small talk were as impaired as mine. Then, as if trying to spare us the pain of an awkward situation, she turned and pulled me into a long, very loving embrace. In her arms there was no confusion. We loved each other, and whatever else was happening between us would not be able to destroy what we shared in an embrace.

I took a hot tub and caught her at the tail end of lunch.

"I have to leave in five minutes," she said. "Uray and I have a room to clean."

I sat down. Anne began to tell me a story about a guru in San Francisco—how he had discouraged one of his students who idolized him. She left before I had a chance to tell her I didn't think of her as a guru. Nor did I idolize her.

Tuesday night's dinner was in the same vein as lunch. I ate with my group and we celebrated a birthday. Anne was across the room in the lounge talking with friends. When we finished our cake, I walked over to see her. She smiled warmly and made room for me on her pillow.

"Here, sit down," she said, "but I have to leave in two minutes."

She introduced me to the woman across from us, then with a burst of energy took me into her arms. I put my head on her chest and wrapped my arms around her waist, and in a surge of love that felt as though it lit our corner of the room, my disappointment vanished.

I was wondering what the woman across from us must be thinking when I was pulled in by a sound that made the room disappear. Against Anne's chest I began to hear the deep purring of small, subtle, pleasure moans that stopped as she inhaled and released with her breath.

I lost myself in her rhythm. The love between us was so exquisite my body no longer felt structured. And then, as I softly pulled in on her waist, I began to perceive it as my own; my ego boundary was gone and we were no longer separate. I was holding my own soft, rounded, compassionate soul — feeling its bliss, listening to its pleasure — its satisfaction that I had returned.

"This feels like home," I said.

She squeezed me tightly, then whispered in my ear, "Uray's standing over there waiting for me. I'm sorry. I have to go."

I sat up and said good-bye. Still feeling the sweet satisfaction of knowing, that no matter what else happened that week, I had given and received the embrace I had longed for. And I felt it in every fiber in my body.

I walked back to my group with Catherine and Paul. We stopped by the message board, as I saw one with my name.

> *Live each present moment completely and the future will*
> *take care of itself.*
> *Love,*
> *Jill*

We had a good session that night: Terry led an anger workout that became pretty intense, then he cranked up some Springsteen and we all started to dance. We were wound up until midnight — didn't return to our room until one.

At 2:00 a.m., Catherine lifted her head off her pillow. "You're not asleep, are you?"

"I'm not even tired," I said.

We talked until sunrise, then fell asleep for an hour.

It was Wednesday morning and, I went in for breakfast. Anne walked in about the time I was finished. She sat down alone. I poured some tea, sat next to her and put my arm around her shoulder, hoping the touch would somehow ground me. She tensed with a hint of annoyance, dug her fork into her boiled egg and twisted out the yolk. I struggled to decide which would be more awkward – getting up and leaving or staying next to her. A man from her group came up and sat down. She introduced us, and left.

I passed Uray on the path twice that day. He glared at me out of the corner of his eye, like a little boy guarding the border of a hostile land. I wanted to slap him. Tell him he was about as intimidating as a bug on the bottom of my shoe. But I didn't need to add to the tension, so I ignored him and went about my day. The hours were now passing slowly. I assumed Anne was still planning to meet me that night, so I spent the afternoon down on the beach, telling myself that whatever was happening with her was about her, and not about me.

I ate dinner that night with some people from my workshop, spending the meal poking at my food. Anne walked in with Uray. They filled their plates and sat down across the room. I couldn't stand the wait, so I asked Paul for his towel and got up to go to the hot tubs. I walked up to Anne to tell her where I'd be, but before I could open my mouth she snapped, "Do you mind. We're eating. I'll meet you when we're finished."

Her tone was so harsh, I felt like I'd been slapped in the face.

"I just wanted to ask what time we were meeting so I could go down to the hot tubs."

She looked at her watch. "I'll meet you back here in forty-five minutes."

I walked out in a daze. I wasn't sure what God had in mind when He sent me to her, but I sure didn't deserve to be treated that way.

I went down and sat in the tubs. Twenty minutes later Uray walked in, took off his clothes and took the furthest hot tub from me. I assumed he was to be my sign that Anne was ready. I stayed in the hot springs for another twenty minutes.

I walked back to the cafeteria and sat down next to Catherine. Anne walked up a few minutes later.

"Are you ready?" she said.

"Yes."

I felt as though I was going to a showdown, neither of us talking as we walked out on to the lawn and down to a pair of large rocks.

Anne sat on one while I sat on the ground and leaned against the other.

"What is going on with you?" I asked.

"What do you mean?"

"The push pull. One minute you love me, the next minute you want me to get the hell out of here."

She nodded. "I admit there has been some of that, but that's because I didn't know what kind of relationship I wanted to have with you when you left here. But I have clarity now, and when you leave here on Friday, I want to say good-bye to you."

"That's fine."

"It is?

"Yes, it is. Anne, I have a husband and three children to go home to. I didn't come up here to try and attach myself to you. And to tell you the truth, I hadn't even thought about what our relationship would be like when I left here."

She looked confused. "When you said the other night that you were never going to lose me again, it sounded like you had thought about it."

"What I'm never going to lose again is what I saw in you. And I needed to hear myself say that. What kind of relationship we have when I leave here seems to be irrelevant to why I'm here."

"Then I should probably back up. Why are you here?"

I set back my shoulders. "I told you. I got the message to go to where you were. That we were to spend time together. That it was time to heal your heart and that when the light came through you to me, I was supposed to give it back to you. Anne, I didn't take this path, this path took me."

"I don't buy that. We all hear many voices. It was your choice to act on them."

"No, Anne, it is not the voice you think. I'm not a child anymore."

"I'm not so sure about that."

I glared at her.

"That didn't come out right," she said. "I mean to the extent that none of us really grow up. I mean we all have stuff left over from our childhood. I know I do, and I know most of my friends do."

That was obvious.

"I know the information I received was real. I didn't make it up," I said.

"I didn't say you did. But that sounded a little like you were trying to convince yourself."

I thought the frustration was going to split my head open. Throughout my journey, it was the closest I had come to feeling as though I was truly going to lose my mind. I pulled at the roots of my hair and stared up at the sky, the stars twinkling their message. *Steady, steady, steady, all is well, as it's supposed to be.*

"What's with the hair pulling? she asked.

I stood up and snapped at her. "Why did God have to set me up with you? Why couldn't Jesus have come into my life? He's dead. He would have been easy to love. It's people that are a fuckin' nightmare, and loving you hasn't been easy."

She chuckled.

"More times than once I've wanted to rip you from my heart and get you the hell out of my life," I said.

"I know the feeling."

"But I knew I had to keep loving you. No matter what, I just had to keep loving you."

"But I keep hearing you say you want something from me. That you're trying to get something that I don't want to give."

"No, Anne, I told you that I knew this was my own experience."

She paused for a moment. "When is your workshop over?" she said.

"Friday at noon."

"I break for lunch at noon," she said. "I'll meet you in the cafeteria. But if what is supposed to happen between us doesn't happen by then, I still want to say goodbye to you."

"That's fine. I want to be free of this relationship as much as you do."

"Dawn, I'm already free of this relationship. And I don't think you understand that."

I nodded in disgust. *You might be free of me. But you're not free.*

She stood up to leave while I struggled to make sense of her ambivalence. "What were your transferences again?" I asked.

She looked annoyed. "I told you that the other day."

"Well, tell me again."

"I took you for a daughter."

There was more going on here than that. "Was this ever sexual for you?"

· "No. Never."

"Then I don't know what your problem is," I said. "But I want you to know that I have never idolized you, and I have never thought of you as a guru. As far as I'm concerned, you're just as screwed up as I am."

She started to laugh, which softened the moment. I took a deep breath and calmed myself down.

"Anne, I know I dumped a bunch of stuff on you the other day in the hot tubs, but my intentions in coming here were pure."

She nodded. "This has been really hard for me, but I feel better now." She put her hands in her pocket, keeping her distance, trying to prove her point.

"I gather this means you can't hug me anymore," I said.

She opened her arms, her embrace rigid and cold. The night before I'd been taken to heaven. Tonight the gates were closed.

I turned on my flashlight and we walked up the grass.

"I'm glad we got this settled," she said, "because I came here to work on another relationship and I really need to move on to those issues."

I shook my head and laughed at myself. I had been a fool for love. A tenacious, incorrigible fool.

"What's so funny?" she asked.

"Nothing. Nothing at all."

She asked me to walk her up the hill so she could use my flashlight to see the lock on her bike.

"Fridays are really busy around here," she said as she turned the combination. "I'll check my schedule, but, I'm only going to have about twenty minutes to meet with you."

"Whatever, Anne. Whatever."

I left Anne and went back to the hot springs. There was nobody in the tubs and the tranquillity was comforting. I took off my clothes and stepped in the farthest one out on the patio, floating in the water looking up at the sky. The stars looked so peaceful I wanted to join them, become a light shining down on the drama, no longer a participant, simply an observer.

One of our workshop leaders, Terry, stepped into the hot tubs.

"What are you doing out here alone?" he said.

"Just looking at the stars."

We talked about hiking, the workshop, and Esalen. I didn't need to talk about Anne. I was hurt, but I wasn't devastated.

By the time I got back to my room, my apathy had worn off and anger had set in. Who the hell did she think she was, talking to me like a condescending parent, shoving me to the side so she could get on to something more important? I tossed and turned until Catherine walked in.

"How did it go?" she said.

"I hate her."

"That bad, huh?"

"Yes, that bad." I told her what happened. Or at least my version of it.

"Why do you think she slammed down a boundary like that?" she asked.

"Who knows."

"Why don't you ask her?"

I grabbed a pillow and held it over my lap. "No. I told her I fell in love with her, and I think she thinks I want something from that."

"Do you?"

"I just wanted to be in the love long enough to ground it in myself. And I think that was happening."

Catherine put on her nightshirt. "You were doing the right thing," she said. "I work with teenagers, and the whole trick with them is to hold them steady within the boundaries while we give them a safe place to love. It sounds like Anne did that with you. It's too bad she couldn't follow it through."

I put my pillow back and lay down again.

"As an adult," Catherine said, "what did your mother do when you told her about the abuse?"

My mother was so far from my mind that I had to reach to the archives to remember what she looked like. "She was supportive at first. Then she told me she couldn't give me what I needed, became defensive, and pretty much ended our relationship."

Catherine looked over at me. "It sounds like you found your mother again."

I was so angry I didn't sleep until dawn. I woke up at eight, and went to the cafeteria for breakfast. Anne was sitting at a table alone. I poured myself some tea and walked up to her.

"There are a few things about last night that I would like to clear up," I said.

"Okay."

I sat down across from her. "I know you have felt invaded by me," I said.

"You're right, I have."

"But my intentions in coming here were pure. I really did come here for a higher purpose, and I was achieving it. And if you could just have held me steady, I would have gotten it."

"Gotten what?"

My jaws started to clench. "I would have gotten it. I would have understood the reflection. But instead, you took something I said, created a threatening situation for yourself and pushed me away.

Anne, you're looking for a way out of our conversations before I even have a chance to enter them. You..."

"Stop." She put up her hand. "I would appreciate it if you kept this to your own experience. You don't need to take care of me or try to get involved in my issues."

"Fair."

"Fair? What does fair mean?" she said.

"It means I see where I have done that and you're right, I need to keep this to my own experience of you and not think about what's happening inside of your head."

"Good, that makes me feel a lot better. And you might ask yourself why you feel the need to do that. I need to get some toast, you want some?"

"No, thanks."

She walked over to the toaster. The question was valid. I needed to address why I tried to enmesh our experiences. She came back and sat down.

"I don't have an answer," I said, "but I'll work on it today."

She nodded.

I continued, "I've been thinking about something you said last night, and I would like to leave you with something to think about."

"Okay."

"I know you'd like to get on with your issues with Otto, but you might find you're looking a gift horse in the mouth. If you addressed the issues you have with our relationship, you might find it brings profound clarity to your others."

She looked as though she'd been hit by the obvious.

I stood up and walked away. "See you later."

She turned toward me and slowly waved me a kiss, and for an instant her eyes went lucid, lit up like reflections of the northern star with a love so powerful, an intelligence so far surpassing her own that it looked as though God had incarnated to say: *Congratulations, you made it.*

I walked out bewildered, in awe of what I had just seen, befuddled by being ping-ponged between two extremes. I ran into my roommate crossing the bridge, and the moment our eyes met, I burst into tears. The ping-pong landing on the side of the rejection. I felt so unwanted all I could do was sob.

"That's right," she said as she held me tight. "Just let it go, Dawn. Just let it go."

I don't know how long I cried. At one point I tried to pull away, but she sensed I wasn't finished and pulled me closer. At least three more waves of tears rose up from my chest as she firmly rubbed my back, pushing the energy up my spine. When I finished, she held my shoulders and looked into my eyes.

"Life ain't for sissies," she said.

I started to laugh. "You got that right."

I went back to the big house and found one of the workshop leaders, Gina, sunning herself on the patio. She offered me a seat and I pulled up a chair to face the ocean.

"How's your reunion with your therapist going?"

"Not so good."

"What's going on?"

"I'm not really sure."

"Let me rephrase that," she said. "What are your perceptions of what's going on?"

I looked out at the water. "I think she wants to feel the love, but I also think she feels invaded by me. And I think she feels that if she gives in to the love, I'm going to try to take something she doesn't want to give."

"And if perception is reflection, can you see where that may apply to you?"

I thought about it and put it in the first person. "I want to feel the love, but I don't want to be invaded. And I'm afraid if I give in to the love, it's going to take something I don't want to give."

Damn, I was watching what I do with the Christ light.

"Yes," I said, "I can see where I do this."

"And if you could tell the part of you that you see in Anne what your intentions were, what would you say?"

"I don't want to possess you. I just want to love you."

And such was the truth of the Christ light.

I turned toward Gina. "But there is another dynamic here. There is a part of me that wants to take care of her. She might be sensing that as a trap. And maybe it is."

"Why do you feel the need to take care of her?"

"I don't know. I guess I'd feel more secure if she needed me, if somehow our experiences were enmeshed."

She nodded. "You know, when children get their boundaries blown open like you had as a child, it's hard to know where you end and somebody else begins. We enmesh with people to comfort a fear."

"What's the fear?"

She smiled. "I don't know, what is it?"

I closed my eyes and pulled it up from the dull pain lingering in my stomach. "I don't want to be abandoned. Not again."

She put her arm around me. "Then don't leave your self."

We had the afternoon off, and Paul, Catherine and I went for a hike. We followed the creek into the forest on a red-powdered trail that had worn from the clay. On the edge was a deep green moss that ran through beds of ferns and up the trunks of redwoods. We crossed over a log and walked up the other side where the creek began to pool in large ponds up the path. Paul pointed out the wildlife, doing his best to keep me in the present. Catherine rubbed my shoulders occasionally but let me walk in silence.

I don't buy that. We all hear many voices. It was your decision to act on it. Anne's words ran through my head a hundred times. She didn't believe me. The woman who showed me faith and spirit had lost her faith in me. I choked off my tears half a dozen times, kept my eyes on the path and tried to keep moving.

"Look at that tree slug," Paul said. He grabbed a stick and tried to pry the bright yellow creature off the tree.

Not long ago, I would have helped him; now I pleaded with him to let it be. He smiled at me and left it alone. We hiked for a couple of hours, then walked back down for dinner. I ate fast and left. I didn't want to see Anne until it was time to say good bye.

The Thursday night workshop was held in the hot tubs. On the way to the session I passed by the message board, opened the one with my name on it.

> *Love is the power through which all things are united.*
> *Love, Jill.*

Catherine walked up, and we went down to the hot springs. The group was assembling for what Terry and Gina called an Esalen Indian cleansing ceremony. Nobody was really sure what that meant, but it required all twenty-four of us to strip naked, shower, then meet in a private room on the south side of the baths where two large tubs where being prepared. We laughed amongst ourselves as we gathered; what was about to happen wasn't going to translate well back in our suburban lives and white collar jobs.

When we entered the room, we paired up around two massage tables. The tables were piled with coarsely — ground salt that our partners were to rub on our skin to cleanse our body of any outer impurities. Catherine and Paul worked on me, then we switched, showered and went to the next step. A table piled with cornmeal was rolled into the room, and, laughing like children taking a mud bath, we took handfuls of cornmeal and covered our bodies.

We showered again and lined up around a large, Roman-style tub where a sacred aromatic oil was dropped into the water for cleansing and a dozen candles were lit around the rim. Terry gestured for silence as we all climbed into the tub; following his lead, each of us came to the center and submerged for a re-birthing.

When the silence was broken, we sang, chanted, laughed and re-birthed. And at midnight, when there didn't seem to be an ounce of impurity left in my body, Paul walked me back to the Big House, and I poured myself into bed.

In the morning, I was awakened by a warm sensation in my chest. I rolled over, and just before I opened my eyes, I saw a flash of soft, white light that looked as though it had pushed through a vertical opening in my heart.

I am faith and spirit.

I opened my eyes, feeling like a child awakening on Christmas morning. I was faith and spirit. I had taken the path, believed in the love, stayed devoted to my heart. Me. I did it. I was the voice of faith in my head, the spirit that had showed me compassion, the guidance that had always been with me.

And in that moment, I realized I was not separate from God, but part of Him. A branch on His tree, a ray from His sun. Connected, loved and accepted for everything I was, everything He created me to be.

I jumped out of bed and into the shower, rested my head against the wall while the hot water ran down my back. It was my faith that had taken me to Esalen. It was my faith and spirit that had survived my childhood. It was me, I was what I had been looking for.

I burst into tears and started to quiver. *Thank you, God. Thank you, thank you, thank you.*

I got out of the shower, wiped the steam off the mirror and looked into my eyes. And I was there, I was me, and I knew who that was.

I dressed and walked down to the living room, grabbed a pen and paper and wrote a note to Anne.

> *I got it:*
> *I am faith and spirit.*
> *Thank you, Dawn*

I missed her at breakfast, but we were saying goodbye at lunch, so I put the note in my pocket and went in for our final group.

We sat in our sacred circle, happy to be going home, sad to be leaving each other. There was a pile of small crystals in the center of the room. Terry asked each of us to take a stone and share with the group what we were taking from Esalen.

I went first, picking up a stone and turning to the group. "I'm taking trust. And I trust that I'm always where I'm supposed to be. With the people I'm supposed to be with. Thank you all very much for helping me through this week."

A few people went after me, then Paul came to the center of the circle. "I'm taking a new appreciation for life," he said. He turned and gestured toward me. "And I fell in love."

I felt a warm flush come up from my chest as his words brought a large part of my heart back into light. It was okay to fall in love. For my heart to come alive with the thought of another person. I put my hands together and bowed.

"Thank you, Paul. Thank you."

We took pictures and exchanged addresses, then I said my goodbyes to the group and put my bags into my car. I walked through the gardens and picked up the path to the cafeteria. Passing the message board, I saw a picture of me. I spun on my heels and walked up to a poster on the board as large as the board itself. I stepped closer. It was a collage of my family with a note from Philip asking Esalen to post it on the board.

I pulled it down, tears streaming from my eyes. There was a picture of Samantha and me on the day she was born. *Life's pain can turn into Life's pleasures...* was written underneath in Philip's handwriting. Next to it was a picture of Maxx running in the water. *Never quit chasing your dreams...* In the corner was a picture of Michael asleep in the bottom of an empty swimming pool. *Peace is where you find it...*

I scanned the collage for a picture of Philip and found him in a photo with the kids. *We are your family* was written underneath. I looked at his image, and my heart came alive at the sight of him.

There were twenty pictures, all with captions, and each one made me miss my family more. I took the poster into the cafeteria and sat down on a bench. There was a picture of the kids all sitting on a curb. They looked so big. Erica was almost as tall as Michael, and I couldn't remember the day she grew up, the first time I heard her talk, or saw her walk or crawled across the floor.

Anne walked up, looking to the buffet line and then back at me. I showed her the collage and then went to get a glass of water. When I returned, she was smiling, more present.

"Phil sent this to you?" she said.

"Yes, he and the kids must have made it after I left."

We talked about a few of the pictures. I was proud to show them off.

"Fridays are really busy here," she said. "I only have about fifteen minutes."

"That's all right, it won't take that long."

I picked up my poster, and we walked down to the rocks.

"You look happy," she said.

"I am. You weren't the only person I was supposed to meet here."

"I'm glad to hear that." She sounded relieved. "Do you want to share?"

I looked at her, and a few feet in front of me I suddenly felt the edge of my own boundary. I knew where I ended and she began. I was whole within myself. There was no need to share.

"No," I said. And it felt so good, I said it again. "No."

She nodded and smiled.

"Well, good-bye," I said.

"That's it? You're ready?"

"Yes, I finally figured it out. I got it this morning."

"It? You keep saying that. What is it?"

I reached in my pocket and handed her the note.

> *I got it:*
> *I am faith and spirit*
> *Thank you, Dawn*

She read it and shivered. "This gives me goose bumps," she said.

"It gave me goose bumps, too. But this morning, I woke up into it. A flash of light came through my heart and I got it—I realized completely, throughout my whole body that what I saw in you was really in me. This was about me, about my journey, about trusting myself and my path. It was my faith that brought me here and it was my faith that I would see you again. I am what I saw in you, Anne. And I'll never lose that again."

"I don't really know what to say."

"It's just like the Wizard of Oz," I said. "You travel to Oz to find out that what you were looking for, you had all along. All you had to do was use it."

"And you have to go to the witch's castle and deal with the flying monkeys," she said.

"Yeah, and the power to go home was with you all along."

We stood up from the rocks and she handed me the note. "Here, do you want this back?"

"No. It's for you to keep. I'm at peace with our relationship."

"You are?"

"Yes, I am." I didn't know why, but I was.

I reached over and hugged her.

"Thanks for being my mom," I said.

"You were a good daughter," she replied. "And you make one hell of a woman."

We pulled apart. "You were a good love object to see that in."

She smiled. "I'm glad to hear you say that, because I have something for you, and I wasn't sure how you would receive it. It's a poem that was given to me in a workshop here. I've kept a copy for me, and I made a copy for you. I know it's something I need to keep in mind."

We walked back to the cafeteria, and she pulled a piece of paper out of her backpack. I opened it up and read it in front of her.

LOVE AFTER LOVE

THE TIME WILL COME
WHEN, WITH ELATION,
YOU WILL GREET YOURSELF ARRIVING
AT YOUR OWN DOOR, IN YOUR OWN MIRROR,
AND EACH WILL SMILE AT THE OTHER'S WELCOME
AND SAY, SIT HERE. EAT.
YOU WILL LOVE AGAIN THE STRANGER WHO WAS YOUR SELF.
GIVE WINE. GIVE BREAD. GIVE BACK YOUR HEART
TO ITSELF, TO THE STRANGER WHO HAS LOVED YOU
ALL YOUR LIFE, WHOM YOU HAVE IGNORED
FOR ANOTHER, WHO KNOWS YOU BY HEART.
TAKE DOWN THE LOVE LETTERS FROM THE BOOKSHELF,
THE PHOTOGRAPHS, THE DESPERATE NOTES,
PEEL YOUR OWN IMAGE FROM THE MIRROR.
SIT. FEAST ON YOUR LIFE.

— From, Collected Poems by Derek Walcott —

I went back in her arms and started to cry. She still felt closed. I felt completely alive and open. "I got it," I said. "I got it."

She put on her backpack, and placed her fist over her heart. "You're always here."

I gestured the same. "Always."

"Goodbye, friend."

"Goodbye, Anne." I picked up my poster and headed home.

When I pulled out of Esalen, I was overcome by elation. It was the first time I realized my mission was complete. I had received the light and given it to Anne. All she had to do was accept it — open the note and say to herself:

> *I got it:*
> *I am faith and spirit.*
> *Thank you, Dawn.*

And when she owned it for herself, she would thank me. And the rejection I had felt from her throughout the week melted into a blissful satisfaction. *We don't really know who people are* — and it applied to me, too.

I stopped in San Luis Obispo to have dinner with my brother. It had been a year since our last dinner together. Steve and Mark, the two men with whom we had eaten, had both since died from AIDS. Their suffering felt even more tragic. Yet, strangely, it no longer frightened me.

James and I drove downtown to pick up a pizza, and at a stop sign, just on the outskirts of town, my chest began to warm and Anne's voice came through my heart. *I got it. I got it.*

In the weeks that followed Esalen, I found myself in a new process. I grieved the fantasy I had lost in Anne, as I welcomed the truth in myself, chiming myself back to wholeness by releasing the same small, subtle, pleasure moans that I heard against Anne's chest. The sound brought the deep love and comfort of my own spirit back into my awareness.

I now knew the Light existed in me, as it does in all, and while I cannot explain the mystery behind it, I had a childhood memory one night that made me realize what the Christ light meant to me.

It was a few nights before Christmas. I had just put the girls to bed and was walking past Michael's room when I felt a comfort in the air inviting me to enter. Michael was asleep. I pulled the covers around his chin and lay down under the quilt on the other bed. The peaceful presence in the room, the smell of fresh pine and the feel of being in a twin bed took me back to my fifteenth year, the Christmas Eve after my friend Joyce died. My friend Sue had picked me up in her mother's old, blue station wagon and had taken me to midnight Mass in the Catholic church across from my elementary school.

When the carols began, we squeezed in through the side door and stood against the wall in the back. The song was Silent Night, and as I sang along, my chest warmed with a deep sense of love, an assurance of peace.

As I recalled that evening, I realized that the Light had always been with me. In my joy, through my suffering, guiding me through my relationship with others, teaching me what the child in the manger came to teach us all — our capacity to love: with all our hearts, with all our minds, and with all our souls.

Epilogue

This month marks the third year since my week at Esalen. It has been a quieter time to assimilate the experiences in my life and the spiritual energy that flows through my body. In many ways this makes me feel different. Life is more peaceful, my relationships more intimate, and my sense of taste, touch and smell are far more vivid.

Yet, along with these moments of calm and self-acceptance, there have also been grave disappointments. My parents have not returned into my life. I understand this, at least with regard to my father, to be a permanent arrangement. But even greater than this loss, was the loss in my belief that enlightenment would cure me from past experiences. Unfortunately, that belief was not true. As a human, I fall, again and again. I have spiraled back to old patterns of fear. I have tapped and again experienced self-destructive emotions. And, on occasion, I still have flashbacks of sexual abuse.

Although these times of regression have been difficult, they continue to decrease in intensity and duration, and I move through them with an expanded awareness that teaches me a better way to live. In other words, I am still work in progress, learning the discipline it takes to stay aligned with my soul, learning the lessons behind my experiences as I live out my life as a wife, a mother, a friend, and a writer.

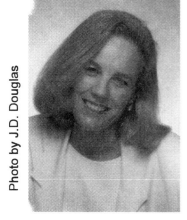

About the Author

Dawn Kohler was the co-founder and President of Icon Computer Corporation, a personal computer service company supporting the Southern California Area. When her company sold in 1994, Dawn pursued her interests in self-healing and psychology. She is now a speaker and workshop leader on the issues of psychological healing, sexual abuse and the signs and symptoms of spiritual transformation. Dawn is currently working on her second book in the self-help/spiritual genre. She lives in Orange County with her husband and three children.

If you would like more information about the book, author speaking engagements or workshops, please contact us at:

www.dawnrising.com